WHAT IS THE BEST ESSENTIAL OIL COMPANY?

Cutting Through The Lies

Bill Liebich

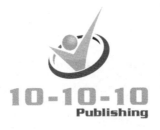

10-10-10
Publishing

What Is The Best Essential Oil Company? Cutting Through The Lies

TheBestEO.com

First 10-10-10 Publishing Paperback Edition June 2019
Second 10-10-10 Publishing Paperback Edition June 2019

Publisher
10-10-10 Publishing
Markham, ON Canada

Printed in Canada and the United States of America

Table of Contents

Acknowledgements

To my beloved wife **Carrie Liebich**, the love, encouragement, support and sacrifice that you have given in making this book happen mean the world to me. I am so very thankful to have you in my life, to be with you while going through this journey together. You are a constant source of joy to me, and I am grateful that you said "Yes" almost two decades ago. You do an incredible job raising our eight children, and I love you and appreciate all that you do every day!

To my wonderful children, **Ezekiel**, **Abigail**, **Bethany**, **Rebekah**, **Jubilee**, **Malachi**, **Hosanna**, and **Solomon**, you are a constant source of joy, laughter and fun. I enjoy watching you explore life, learn new skills, master difficult tasks, and figure out solutions. I'm amazed at the care, love and support you show for your brothers and sisters and your willingness to help. You are the reason I began this journey to find the best essential oils in the world and would never settle for less. Your health and quality of life are that important to me! I love each and every one of you and I am proud of you!

To my parents, **Roger** & **Rosemary Liebich**, thank you for the love, care, training, guidance, and support you have given me! I appreciate the faith in Christ that you instilled in me and your continued prayers for my well-being and success. With gratitude I recognize all the schooling that you selflessly paid for and the ways that you sacrificed to enable me to grow and learn. Thank you for helping me always do better, push myself, and not give up. I love you!

To my brothers, **Jim** and **Brian**, thank you for the competition. That seems like a weird thing to be thankful for, but someone needed to teach me, "never give up, never surrender, and the battle is never over." You've helped me hone my stubbornness into steadfastness and I will be forever grateful to you for that.

To **David & Georgeann Wellfare** and **Don & Arlene Kent**, thank you for welcoming me into your family, and making me feel like I belonged from the start! I recognize the little things you have always done to make me feel special, encourage me, and make me feel at home. I always enjoy and look forward to our time together. Your encouragement, positivity, and belief in me about this book have meant a great deal to me.

To the **Addlemans, Camerons, Charmichaels, Foxes, Franklins, Goodales, Hathaways, MacDonalds, Pereanus, Radtkes, Snymans, Squires, Thornbergs, Villas, Wilfords, Brenden O'Meara**, and the rest of **my Church Family at Cornerstone Bible Church**, thank you for praying for me and my family, asking me about my book's progress, testing my knowledge and abilities, and being a source of encouragement.

To my friends, **John Brock, Bethany Brown, Dawn & Chris Brownwell, John Buffington, Troy & Wendy Cameron, Ben & Marissa Christensen, John & Betsy Clark, Donna Cettolin, Gordon & Corie DeVries, Matt & Shaun Ditty, Daniel Espy, Paul & Kelowna Guiliano, Jennifer Holland, Jonathan Hopkins, Max & Karen Hopkins, Kevin & Heidi Hovan, Randy & Diane Jenkins, Darren & Sera Johnson, Adaryll Jordan, Beth Keifat, Tami Lewis, Brian & Skyla Mann, Allan & Cristina Margate, Michael & Carrie McVige, Roy Mertz, Meg Paulson, Grady & Pat Pennell, Nathan Petty, Naomi Phillips, Jon & Katie Reeves, Brent &**

Sarah Reimers, **Reuben & Amanda Rog**, **Matt Schroepfer**, **Gabe Uribe**, **Rick & Cheryl Vandegrift**, thank you for your friendship, your trust, explanations, prayers, concerns, joys, and knowledge. All of these things are what keep me moving on when I have had hard times and I appreciate your questions, stories, and encouragements that made this book a reality.

To **Amanda Uribe**, thank you for being willing to share with us in the hospital what you had learned. You changed our lives that night, and our family is eternally grateful for your courage and your gifts. Every time Jubilee smiles, it is possible because you cared. Lastly, I really appreciate your research and knowledge on what you shared on toxins. Overall, this book never would have happened if it hadn't been for you to start us on this new paradigm!

To **Chris Opfer**, thank you for your insights on good, better, best and your willingness to share. I appreciate our conversations, interactions, questions, and your readiness to teach me something new. This book is blessed greatly by your comments and friendship.

To **Sonoma State University**, I appreciate the hours spent writing papers and reports, the time management skills I learned, and the degree that led to me having the skills necessary to write a book.

To **Success Resources America**, thank you for your invaluable teaching and training. I would never have been able to write this book without your instruction!

To **KLOVE Radio**, thank you for your positive, encouraging message and music to soothe my life and soul while working on this book.

To **Family Life Radio** and **Intentional Living with Dr. Randy Carlson**, your music and message has been inspirational to me and motivates me to always be willing to do better in my Christian walk and gave me joy while writing this book.

To **Raymond Aaron**, I will always remember our conversation that convinced me that I needed to write a book. Thank you for the inspiration and encouragement to become an author.

To **Christina Fife** and **Liz Ventrella**, your continued support in helping me through every area of publishing and marketing to get the different pieces done and accomplish my book has been invaluable.

To **Waqas Ahmed**, thank you for the wonderful graphics. My book would not be the same without your work.

To **Naval Kumar**, my personal book architect, thank you for all of the help, care, and direction you have given me to enable this book to become a reality.

Foreword

Are you interested in essential oils, and living a toxin-free lifestyle? If so, *What Is The Best Essential Oil Company?* by Bill Liebich is a must- read!

I first met Bill when I was speaking at a Success Resources America event, and the first thing I noticed was his inquisitive nature, and analytical mind. I can assure you that he has a sincere desire to help you.

I was impressed with his knowledge of essential oils; I could tell that he really knew his subject well. It was apparent that he had spent a great deal of time researching the different brands, methods, testing and characteristics of essential oils.

All of this has resulted in *What Is The Best Essential Oil Company*? providing you with an informative look at essential oil companies.

His ability to pick out the smallest details has enabled him to cut through the lies surrounding the essential oil marketplace and present the material to you in a clear, well thought out matter. I am thoroughly impressed with the way Bill covers all the areas of concern and enables you to make the best choice. He provides methods, strategies and questions for you to identify the best essential oils and toxin-free products for yourself.

I highly recommend Bill, and *What Is The Best Essential Oil Company*?

Raymond Aaron
New York Times Bestselling Author

Introduction

In the last few years essential oils have gained market awareness. Instead of mentioning essential oils and getting the blank stare, most people have at least heard about essential oils, even if they don't know a lot about them.

Essential oils are:
- Found in plants, trees, and shrubs
- Necessary to the life of that plant
- Aromatic liquids that escape easily into the air
- Sent by plants to a site of disease, infection, injury, and reproduction
- Tested & verified by scientific study to contain many therapeutic properties
- Listed in the Bible and many ancient texts with documented uses

With a little bit of research you can figure out what essential oil company I support. But before you let that make your decision for you, I'd like you to keep an open mind and ask yourself and your essential oil company the points, thoughts and questions that I bring up.

As I began my journey into essential oils more than 6 years ago, I did a lot of research to make sure I was getting the best essential oils for my family. I analyzed the propaganda, the different companies found in the grocery store and even the Network Marketing/Multi- Level Marketing companies.

I wanted the best quality essential oils for my family and I have shared that knowledge with others throughout the years. It is my sincere desire for you to have a greater understanding of what factors to look for to choose the best essential oil company.

With numerous brands of essential oils on the market, with varying years of time in business and with multiple methods and types of distillation, how can any one company say that they are the best company? Even worse, with no regulating body for the strength, quality, purity or grade of essential oil, every company can say whatever they want about themselves.

So I ask you to keep an open mind, ask your own essential oil company the questions you will find as you read through this book, and examine their responses. I hope you find the answers you seek in this book and that you are able to find the best essential oil company.

I hope you have a wonderful time reading this book and have a blessed day!

Bill Liebich

Dedication

I dedicate this book to my children.
Let this book always be a reminder to write down
your goals and reach for them. Hold onto my
belief in you until you believe in yourselves.
When you believe in yourself, don't give up,
and don't settle for less than the best,
you will not only reach your dreams,
you will leave a legacy!

CHAPTER 1

Propaganda – The Lies People Tell

*"Truth is the ultimate power. When the truth comes
around, all the lies have to run and hide."*
~Ice Cube

A Simple Look At The Bottle

When looking to cut through the propaganda to get the best oils, one of the most important tools to use is to look at what the company says about themselves. The first way is to just simply look at the bottle, and read the label. What will a simple look at the bottle tell you about quality vs. worthless junk? Well, let's dive in and find out!

Does the bottle contain any warnings about breathing the oil or applying it to your skin? Are there any poison warnings or ingestion warnings? A pure essential oil is simply that, a pure extract from the plant itself. It should not need warnings for application or smelling. Do you get warnings when you go to a nursery? "Don't smell the flowers." The whole concept is ridiculous! Let's look at Peppermint, Lavender and Rose essential oils. For consistency's sake, I am going to refer to Peppermint, Lavender and Rose essential oils repeatedly in this book. These plants are safe to touch (not the rose thorns!), smell and eat, so the essential oils made from these plants should also be safe to touch, smell and ingest. In the world of essential oils that corresponds to the 3 methods of use: touch = topical use, smell = aromatic use, and ingest = internal use.

If you go out into the field, pick a leaf off a peppermint plant and rub the leaf between your fingers, you have just used the oil topically. If you smell your fingers, you have just used the oil aromatically, and if you take a bit of the leaf and chew on it, you have just used the oil internally.

So, back to the bottle, if you see warnings about breathing the essential oil, RUN AWAY! Life is too short, why would you want to breathe toxins? Why would you fear smelling a plant?

Next, look at the ingredients list. Is there any alcohol in there, or other chemicals you can't pronounce? I'm not talking about Latin plant names like (Mentha piperita) for Peppermint, (Lavandula angustifolia) for Lavender and (Rosa damascena) for Rose, I'm talking about chemicals. True essential oils should NOT have any chemicals or alcohol added to them. Chemicals and alcohol are signs of shortcuts and cheap quality essential oils. Life is too short; why would you want to apply toxins or settle for lesser quality?

Another thing to look for is the expiration date. There were essential oils found in King Tut's tomb that were still good, and true essential oils shouldn't expire, so what is the reason for the expiration date? If it's not the essential oils that expire it must be something inside the essential oils that is expiring. For instance, maybe they've diluted it with a carrier oil, or polluted it with a synthetic to squeeze even more sales out of the same amount of essential oil.

Diluted –

1. A method of applying essential oils directly to the skin with the use of a carrier oil to slow down the absorption rate of the essential oil. Usually used with "hot" oils to reduce the perceived heat of the oil.

2. A consumer's cost saving method; used to combine a small amount of essential oil with a small amount of carrier oil for the purpose of spreading it over a greater surface area.

3. A deceptive cost saving method, used to combine a small amount of essential oil with a large amount of carrier oil for the purpose of selling a larger amount of a weaker strength essential oil.

Carrier oil – a fatty seed oil like coconut, avocado, sesame or olive oil.

Lastly let's look at the size of the bottles. One of most common methods of trying to make more money from the sale of essential oils is to dilute them with a carrier oil and sell the same amount of essential oil multiple times for a larger profit. A sure sign of a low quality essential oil is that instead of a normal 5 ml or 15 ml bottle you have some giant sized 450 ml or so bottle of Peppermint, Lavender or even Rose being sold for $10. What you're paying for is a diluted essential oil rather than a full strength essential oil. What is even worse is the essential oil that was diluted may have been nothing more than synthetic junk.

Essential Oils Don't Come From A Lab

The chemical structure of an essential oil is something that can be copied and reproduced in a lab, but that doesn't mean that they have the same properties. While the chemical structure of the essential oil moves and twists like it is alive and intelligent, the copy is static, frozen in time. Since the DNA of our bodies is similar to essential oils, our bodies know how to process essential oils, but the copies made from petroleum products are toxic and our bodies do not process them the same way. Petroleum products build up to toxic levels in our bodies and cause major health problems.

To further illustrate that point, I'd like to tell you a story...

A healthy, female, high school track-and-field athlete, while preparing for a track meet, had been using a popular topical sports cream that has synthetic methyl salicylate in it to help with inflammation. Unfortunately, she used too much of the sports cream over a short period time and ended up dying when the methyl salicylate built up to a toxic level in her system.

Our bodies can process pure essential oils. There are also quenching properties in essential oils when you don't dismantle them and take parts and pieces away.

The quenching effect is a process that is well known by today's chemists and manufacturing companies. Soda manufacturers utilize the quenching effect when making soda. The amount of sugar in most soda cans is about 10 teaspoons, and if you were to try to eat that much sugar once your body would throw it up because your body recognizes the danger, but unfortunately thanks to the quenching effect, the acid in the soda makes your body swallow it.

The quenching effect is further continued, when at 20 minutes after you swallow the soda your body would be going into a diabetic coma if it didn't quench the sugar by turning it into fat. The quenching effect continues an hour after drinking the soda by leaching calcium, magnesium and zinc from your bones and body to bond with the sugar, allowing your body to get rid of it as waste.

Pure essential oils are more powerful than their synthetic counterparts and have quenching effects too. Even though the synthetic methyl salicylate used by the topical sports cream was copied from Wintergreen essential oil, the copy is only one part of the whole and therefore contains no quenching effects. It is, however, those same quenching effects that protect you as well.

My friend's mom, Karen, was dropping Wintergreen essential oil under her tongue when unfortunately the orifice reducer came loose and she accidentally poured three-quarters of a 15ml bottle down her throat and swallowed. As essential oils help our bodies to detoxify from chemicals and live even healthier and cleaner lives, it "helped" her push out the toxins very quickly. Needless to say, she needed a bathroom nearby and a bed to rest on for a day until she felt better, but she lived to tell the tale because of the quenching properties of the essential oil.

Finally, take Lavender as an example. There are many more Lavender scented products on the market than there is Lavender essential oil produced in the world. The two biggest problems that happen with Lavender essential oil are that either the manufacturers replace Lavender (Lavandula angustifolia) with Lavandin (Lavandula intermedia) or they make a synthetic copy of Lavender. Lavandin has a similar smell to Lavender, but not the same therapeutic properties. That means that there is a high likelihood that the Lavender scented products you just bought for your kitchen, baby's room, bathroom or even business are probably either synthetic, or Lavandin.

As I've already said, synthetics are bad, but how bad? I could literally write another book on how bad synthetic fragrances are for you. To give you an idea, they are carcinogenic or cancer causing, hormone disruptors, and they damage your organs and cells, cause allergies, headaches, rashes and even death.

Now that we have touched on the nastiness of synthetics, let's talk about smelling essential oils.

Smelling The Difference

Can just smelling the oil tell you anything about its quality? Can you tell by the strength of the scent if it has been diluted? The answer to both questions is yes. Essential oils are much like a fine wine that varies from year to year.

A wine taster or collector will go on and on about how a certain year of wine was better than all the other years because of its sweetness, tartness or how bitter it was. All of these factors are determined by the rainfall, the amount of sunshine, what time of day the grapes were harvested, or even what kind of fertilizer was used.

Essential oils are the same; they vary from plant to plant and even from one side of the field to the other. Take peppermint for instance: you might have a really strong menthol smell in one portion of field, while another might smell more musty like tobacco, and that's just the range of peppermint plant from one field in the same year.

So what does that tell you? If you come across a brand of Peppermint essential oil that smells exactly the same with every bottle, over different batches in different years, you need to question what the manufacturer is doing to that oil to make it smell that way. Are they extracting something from it to make it smell less potent or are they adding something synthetic to it to make it smell sweet like candy? The only way to get a plant-derived product like an essential oil to smell the same every time is to use a synthetic.

Additionally, you can smell Peppermint essential oil from multiple bottles over multiple vendors and start to recognize that certain lines smell really weak, other ones smell stronger, or that one might be candy sweet and still another will be so strong it makes you say, "Whoa!" If the smell is so faint you can barely smell it, then it's probably being diluted.

Before I started using essential oils from my favorite essential oil company, a friend gave me a few fragrance oil vials and a warmer plate to use with them. Dropping the oils onto the warmer plate slowly heats them and releases their fragrance into the air. The warmer was kept in the master bathroom and I used a few drops on the warmer after a smelly event.

Hours later, at bedtime, my wife and I had trouble breathing because the fragrance made our throats itch. I ended up opening up the window in the middle of winter in Alaska to remove the fragrance and allow us to sleep. I have encountered this reaction multiple times since then, and always with synthetic fragrances, from perfumes, synthetic essential oils and from warmers for melting candle wax.

I have an additional warning for you, if you are using candle wax warmers in your home or bedroom. A few years ago, I repainted a room that had been used for some time with a candle wax warmer. The paint would not stick to the top two inches of the wall next to the ceiling from all the candle wax melted in that room.

Within five minutes after applying paint to the top few inches, most of the paint would flow down the wall and leave the top few inches mostly unpainted. Needless to say, it took me a very long time to paint that room. The warning for you is this: if it will leave that much residue on the ceiling line, how much residue is being left in your lungs?

This Is A Plant...Where Are The Farms?

Another question you may want to ask your essential oil company is if they own their own farms, or if they use partner farms that they visit regularly. Why would this be important? Well, if they own their own farms or use partner farms that they visit regularly, they can monitor the process of how the plants are grown and ensure the quality of their plants at distillation. They can also ensure that there are no pesticides, herbicides or chemicals sprayed on their plants. Basically it means they don't have to be a broker because they know where their plants came from and how they were cared for and they don't have to take somebody else's word for it.

Some companies will tell you that they do not know where their farms are located. Some, even if they know the location, won't tell you where they are because they themselves haven't even visited to check the quality, or they don't want you to check. So there's no way they're going to let you even go on a tour of their farm and see the process of distillation. Also, there are companies that have no farm at all but are actually brokers of essential oils, meaning they go to a marketplace and pick up raw materials or pre-distilled essential oils and sell them as their own.

In fact, a prominent store-based seller of essential oils who I'm going to call Company A, posted with pride on their website about how they go to the source to get their essential oils. You watch the Company A person go to a farm in the middle of nowhere, where the farmer himself is doing the distillation in his aluminum still. When done, the farmer places the essential oils into a used 2-liter plastic bottle! Company A also said that they go to the local marketplace and they pick up more of this essential oil from street vendors, and showed a scene from the marketplace where this 2-liter plastic bottle wasn't necessarily the worst container to be used!

To my horror, the video showed three major problems:

- The distillers were local farmers growing and distilling their own plants by unverified means. These essential oils were not able to be verified free of pesticides or other contaminants during the growing process, nor was there any quality check done on the best procedures for harvesting that plant.

- Even worse, the farmer was using an aluminum still. When aluminum is used in cooking, the aluminum leaches from the container and into the food. The same thing happens with the essential oils. There is no way to verify the distillation procedures of the street vendors to ensure the farmer used the proper method.

- The sellers used any used plastic bottle they could find to hold the essential oils. Not only will toxins leach from the plastic into the essential oils, but so will the residue of whatever the container was used to store previously.

What other store-based, online or network marketing essential oil companies are using this same procedure for bringing you essential oils?

Essential oils are made using agricultural products like plants, trees, roots, resins, bark and leaves. This requires forecasting as much as 6 to 10 years in advance what your demand will be and how much oil you need to have in stock. If your essential oil company never runs out of product and always has their essential oils in stock, then what are they doing to ensure they never run out?

How are they circumventing the forecasting of consumer demand, the amount of raw materials needed and the amount of essential oils those raw materials will produce to meet those demands?

Are they merely brokers of essential oils, finding any supplier necessary to fulfill their quotas and inventory needs? Are they diluting their essential oils to make them last longer and keep them in supply? Are they synthetically creating their essential oils on demand, and not worrying about forecasting a seasonal crop or running out of stock?

If an essential oil company does not know where their farms are, or never runs out of stock, be afraid and run!

My favorite essential oil company would rather run out of an essential oil than compromise on quality. Would you like to count on the quality of your essential oils?

Different Types Of Extraction Or Distillation

Extraction Method – The process of how essential oils are pulled out of plant material.

Solvent Method – Extraction method using a chemical or alcohol to pull out essential oils.

Steam Distillation Method – The cleanest extraction method, using superheated water vapor.

Enfleurage Method – Extraction method using a fatty oil to pull out essential oils.

Pressing Method – Extraction method that uses force to extract essential oils.

Steam distillation is the safest and purest method of extracting essential oils from most types of plant material. The exceptions are that Citrus oils are best when cold-pressed from the rind and there are certain plants like Jasmine and Neroli that do not allow for steam distillation as it destroys the plant material before it releases the essential oils. In that case a solvent, like food grade grain alcohol, must be used.

With steam distillation the plant materials are packed into a large still and steam is slowly allowed to permeate through the layers of plant material where it bonds to essential oils. The essential oil infused steam eventually leaves the still through a hose at the top of the lid, where it goes through a condenser and ends up in a separator where the essential oils automatically float on top of the water. The pure essential oils are taken off the top, leaving the floral water behind as the byproduct.

The floral water contains some of the properties of the essential oil, but is not considered an essential oil on its own.

After helping with the harvest of Idaho Balsam Fir on the farm of my favorite essential oil company, I sat in a Jacuzzi filled with the floral water from an Idaho Balsam Fir Distillation. The water smelled amazing and was very relaxing and soothing to all of my tired muscles and joints.

While I was helping with the harvest, I learned that my favorite essential oil company uses only cone shaped lids on the still, because it lets the steam out right away, instead of making the steam curl around for a while before leaving the still. This produces a higher quality of oil. Additionally, I learned that the stills are made from stainless steel because other metals leach into the essential oils.

A cheaper and easier form of extracting essential oils is to use an Enfleurage-like process through fats, solvents or carrier oils.

Chemical or solvent extraction is the cheapest method of extracting essential oils and is primarily used by the perfume industry, because what is primarily wanted is the scent. There are some botanicals that are too fragile to be extracted via steam distillation and then have to be extracted using grain alcohol. Among these are Jasmine and Neroli.

Two methods of distillation that do not give you the purest or full- strength essential oils are Quick Distillation and Complete Distillation.

With a Quick Distillation, a company does as quick a process as possible to get the scent of the essential oil, but without any reference to the properties of the oil produced. Often this process will be used by a company with an abundance of low quality plant products, and the concern is to minimize the time in the still in order to get the next load through and reduce operating costs.

With a Complete Distillation, the company might have a little knowledge about how to distill essential oils, but has a limited amount of plant material to distill. The company in this case would perform a Quick Distillation, or longer process, over and over again until there is no more essential oil aroma from the plant material. With a Complete Distillation, they combine the first distillation with the following distillations to produce a weaker product.

This is very much like bad and diluted coffee. Most people want a really strong cup of coffee. I assume you'd be offended if you paid full price for a cup of coffee and didn't get what you thought you should. What if the server brewed the coffee and poured it off into a big vat, then ran it again and again and again with the same grounds until the water was clear? What if he took the resulting compilation of coffee and gave you a cup of that coffee? How satisfied would you be? How good would the coffee be?

Ask Yourself...
If you are not okay with a weak cup of coffee, why would you be willing to take a weak bottle of essential oil? Would you prefer a full strength essential oil? Would you prefer to know and trust the method of distillation?

Follow The Money & Motivation

In the essential oil industry, just like in any other business, people follow the money. In this case, starting in 2008 the leading essential oil company experienced exponential growth, and after that new essential oil companies appeared on the market. By 2015, essential oils stopped being just something sold by network marketing companies and health food stores, but something you could find at any department store, warehouse store or even gas station. That, in itself, is not really a surprise, but what is surprising is that the same new companies proclaimed that they were experts in the field.

When I first started with my favorite essential oil company in 2013, most of the competitors in the essential oil marketplace had been around for five years or fewer. At that time, I heard the story of Idaho Balsam Fir essential oil, and how it took 7 years of testing to figure out how to get the greatest amount of therapeutic properties in that essential oil.

The research team had tested various factors, such as time of year to harvest the trees, what part of the tree to use, how best to mulch the tree to increase the surface area and improve contact with steam, what temperature and how long to distill for, and even how tightly to pack the materials for distillation. All of these tests, over 7 years time frame, show a dedication to quality and purity that takes time and experience.

How can a company that's been around for 1 to 5 years really be the expert in the field, when there is a company that has been around for almost 20 years that has documented procedures for creating the best oils? The new companies did whatever they could to try to discredit the larger company and say that they were better. Yet even at the time, there were essential oil companies that had been around for five years or less that thought that they had higher quality essential oils. It's humorous to me that every new company that came on the market claimed that they were better than one particular company.

I think this is humorous because, contrary to what they were saying, their claims actually made that one company stand out as the recognized leader. A true leader in the field doesn't have to declare itself better than anybody else but simply let their quality, effectiveness and integrity stand on its own.

It's also humorous that during that same time frame, "expert" individuals hopped from one company to the next, saying that particular company was now the leader, only to eventually decide they wanted in on the profits and start their own company. Adding to that silliness, when their oils became available, these "experts" claimed they were now the best brand of essential oils.

Another type of motivation I found in websites, blogs and groups was a group I am going to call Group A, who seems to be paid to make it their sole purpose to discredit any form of alternative medicine company, leader or device. Group A has lost many lawsuits for libel, creating false accusations on websites, blogs and letters claiming untruths about leaders of the alternative medical field.

Even though Group A's scandalmongering has been proven many times in court and they have been forced to pay damages, they keep attacking and making comments about leaders, companies, and devices of the alternative medical field. No normal person would continue to lose lawsuits without changing their behavior, without significant funding from somewhere. Group A has attacked the leaders and innovators in the alternative medicine field, including chiropractors, naturopaths, acupuncturists, device manufacturers and even my favorite essential oil company. The motivation seems to be to create a false story to ruin the reputation and livelihood of the person or company.

Because Group A and its leader have been caught so many times, when they attack an alternative medicine leader, business, or device, they are actually validating the importance of that person, company, and device instead of taking away from it.

Going back to motivation, this time spiritual motivation, I have heard many people, when introduced to essential oils, ask the question, "What are the spiritual beliefs of that particular essential oil company?" I find that question to be strange, since I have never heard these same people question their fast-food, computer, appliance, cell phone, furniture, electronic, clothing, grocery store or home supply companies, but suddenly, this question is important to them when dealing with essential oils.

However, the answer is simple. Companies do not have spiritual beliefs, but you can discern the priorities and motivations of their leaders if you follow the money. Where that company spends its money is what is important to that company's leadership. If you truly want to know about a company, check out what causes and charities it supports.

I know where my favorite essential oil company spends its money, and I am very pleased with the ways that they support and care for the abused, mistreated and less fortunate in the world.

Proof In Action – Check The Facts

At the end of each chapter, I will be giving you a list of all the questions I have asked during that chapter for you to question your essential oil company and cut through the lies.

A Simple Look At The Bottle

- Are your essential oils labeled safe to put on the skin? To breathe? To ingest?
- Is there any alcohol or other chemicals in the essential oils?
- Are there any expiration dates?
- What is the reason for the expiration date?
- What size and cost is the bottle? Is it a 5 ml or 15 ml or larger?
- Do you dilute your oils with a carrier oil when bottling?

Essential Oils Don't Come From A Lab

- Are there any synthetics in the essential oils?

Smelling The Difference

- Do the essential oils smell strong or weak?
- Do they smell the exact same way every time?
- Do they smell like the plant or sweet like candy?
- Are you adding something synthetic to the oils to make them smell sweet?

This Is A Plant...Where Are The Farms?

- Do you own your own farms?
- Where are your farms located?
- Can I visit your farms?
- Will there be a guided tour, or can I wander?
- Do you use partner farms that you visit regularly?
- How are weeds removed?
- Are any pesticides or herbicides sprayed on or near the plants?
- What type of fertilizers are used?
- Do any essential oils ever go out of stock?

Different Types Of Extraction Or Distillation

- What type of extraction or distillation method is used?
- Do you sell Rose essential oil? How is it extracted? How much does it cost?
- What shape of lid is used on the still, cone or dome-shaped?
- What type of material is the container made from that is used to distill essential oils?
- Do you use a first distillation or a complete distillation?
- Will you explain your extraction, testing and production process to me?
- Do you have your own facilities for extraction or distillation?
- How many facilities do you have?

Follow The Money & Motivation

- How long has the company been in business?
- How long has the company been working with essential oils?
- When did the company join the essential oil market?
- Where did your company learn how to process essential oils?
- Did you have any training?
- What charities or organizations does your company support?

We have spent some time looking at the Propaganda – The Lies People Tell. I'm hoping that it gave you some food for thought, and questions to ask your essential oil company. In the next chapter, I will be looking at the essential oils available in the grocery store and what standards are used to test these products.

CHAPTER 2

Testing, Standards & Grocery Store Oils

"You figure out what your standards are,
and I think that's important."
~Neil Patrick Harris

Grocery Store Oils

The oils you find in the grocery story are going to fit into one of four categories of varying quality, purity, and manufacture.

First are the essential oils that are fully synthetic, and will say things like do not ingest, do not put on skin and do not inhale. Synthetic means that they are created in a lab, are not natural and are full of toxins. I'm not really sure what these oils are for other than landfill. But so many people are duped into thinking that these are true essential oils and that they are good for them, when in reality, they are making them sick with all the toxins.

The second category of grocery store essential oils is amateur distilling enthusiasts. These are the kind of companies that are started because people think that anyone can make essential oils at home on the stove. In this set of oils, you will find varying quality, varying methods of production and maybe even dilution. Since the people involved in this category have little to no training, they are guessing at methods, times, temperatures, and safety. Often, essential oils in this category have little to no therapeutic value.

The third category is essential oil companies that have been in business for less than 10 years. While some of these companies, with good intentions, have gone for organic certification or some sort of training, and they might have a better quality than some of the amateurs, they still lack the experience in the field and resources to make them truly exceptional. Truly, some of the companies in this category are in the essential oil business to just make money. Often they do not have their own farms, do not have sufficient people to work and monitor the farms, do not do their own distillation, do not test their own oils or even bottle their own oils. On top of all that, the company might just be like Company A that "went to the source" only to buy essential oils in a marketplace that were distilled in an aluminum still and stored in a used plastic bottle.

The fourth category is essential oil companies that have been in the business for 10 or more years. Generally, the companies in this level have learned a thing or two about surviving the startup stage, cutting costs and following the supply chain process. But what is their true dedication to quality? Do they do like Company A that "went to the source?" Do any of them own their own farms? Do they test and bottle their own oils? Do they use synthetics to avoid being out of stock in a product? Do they continually try to improve the quality of their oils? The sad truth is that most of them are still brokers of essential oils, meaning that they get a shipment in, re-label it as their own and send it back out again. Besides my favorite essential oil company, I don't know any of them that own their own farms, cultivate, distill, test, and bottle their own oils.

I have had many friends switch to my favorite essential oil company after just trying a side-by-side comparison of essential oils, because the difference was so drastic and noticeable.

Ask Yourself...

How long has my essential oil company been in business? What were their motives for producing essential oils? How much training do they have in distilling essential oils? How effective are the essential oils you bought at the grocery store? Would you like essential oils that really make a difference?

I Trust The Store Where I Am Buying

While you may have faith in a particular company as a place to find a wide selection of high quality organic and health food products, the company itself is under no obligation to test the essential oils that they have on their shelves. You are simply buying by association; the store is under no obligation to ensure the quality.

Even though the store itself may be known for organic produce or for health food or alternative and hard to find foods, or even generally have the widest selection of products, they themselves have done no testing on and have no requirements for essential oils on their shelves. The store is simply a location for all of the local vendors, and large chain essential oil companies to have a shelf to sell their products. The essential oils are at that store because someone asked the store if they would sell their products. This is not a guarantee that you have the highest quality.

Sometimes the essential oil company is at that store simply because the store decided that they wanted in on the profits from the essential oil industry, or even paid to have their name put on an existing brand. Sometimes that brand of essential oils is on the shelf because they offered a higher percentage of the profits to the chain store if they would carry, advertise and prominently display their brand of essential oils.

Additionally, there is no regulating body for the strength, quality, purity or grade of essential oil. There are an abundance of essential oil companies with varying grades of quality. The types and grades of essential oils are just as varied as the companies that make them. The grades range from perfume grade essential oils full of toxins and synthetic fragrances, to totally pure, therapeutic grade essential oils with better than organic sourcing, testing and standards.

Add to that the fact that not all essential oil companies sell in grocery stores and you have a huge chore in front of you. That means, choosing essential oils based on the stores that sell them is really just a shot in the dark, because you don't even know if the best company is selling in a store. I challenge you to always look at the bottles, compare the processes, call the companies and ask them questions.

Science & Testing

Most companies with essential oils to sell either do so in stores or online, and have little to no testing done on their essential oils. There are few companies that have a fair amount of testing done on their essential oils; however, since people who are exclusively on their payroll do most of the testing, the results show what the company wants them to show.

A true test would involve third party testing, where there is someone from outside the company who is hired to just examine the essential oils and report back the findings. Still, if the third party company doesn't have the expertise to really verify the results, it would not be anything to brag about. In all of these scenarios though, the regimen and types of tests are far too few and mostly basic, especially when compared to the tests run by my favorite essential oil company, which I will cover in Chapter 5.

In some cases, the expertise of the third party labs proves nothing more than they know how to turn on a machine. In fact, not too long ago, a couple of amateur testers accused my favorite essential oil company of having synthetic compounds in their Cinnamon Bark essential oil. The accusation didn't go well for the accusers in the end. Due to my favorite essential oil company's scientists, their vast experience in the equipment used, knowledge of the tests that were run, the extensive library of results and source samples they have produced, and procedures that they stringently follow, the accusation was refuted easily. The scientists were able to share with the accusers where they had gone wrong in their tests, told them how to properly clean the machine between samples, and even what the accusers were testing in their machines beforehand that polluted the results of the Cinnamon Bark essential oil sample. Experience, quality and standards matter!

In a later chapter I will talk much more in depth about what types and amounts of testing are done by my favorite essential oil company. The testing is done multiple times, with multiple stages in the process, by both in-house testing and multiple independent third party testing locations, one of which is the same place that does forensic testing for Scotland Yard.

Would you like your essential oil company to value your health and test your essential oils as thoroughly?

Organic Standards & Regulations

What does "organic standards" really mean? Is there really some sort of governing body that monitors the organic standards for essential oils? No, not really.

The standards themselves were created only for plants and agricultural products, not for essential oils. While the organic certification specifies that the produce and other ingredients are grown without the use of synthetics, sewage, GMOs, ionizing radiation or pesticides that aren't approved organic, it doesn't ensure that the essential oils were extracted correctly, and it only applies to US grown plants and agricultural products. So, if an essential oil company has farms throughout the world, and grows the plants in the native environment, there is no organic certification available.

Did you know the standard to declare a piece of land as organic is only 3 years without pesticides? Pesticide-free for only 3 years! Recently I ran into a woman who did testing on plants in farms that were trying to get their organic certification and she found out from her testing that while the soil itself may not show the pesticides after three years, the plants that were grown in that soil will continue to show the pesticides in them for another 5 years. So wouldn't the better standard be to lengthen that time period to longer than 8 years? Or how about 10 years?

It seems to me that a much better standard would be to lengthen that time period to really be sure that there are no pesticides left in the area or even in the weeds that were in that soil.

A new standard, for better than organic, could be 50 years without pesticides. What if I told you that there is an essential oil company that already uses 50 years without pesticides as their standard for purchasing a farm? This same company won't even consider getting an organic standard because that would mean that they would have to downgrade their standards to organic.

I like working with a company that has better than organic standards, as it allows me to completely trust each and every portion of their process. Doesn't that sound like the kind of company where you would want to shop?

What School Of Thought?

There are three different schools of thought regarding the application and use of essential oils, the British method, the German Method and the French Method.

The British method is a school of thought developed in England, and focuses on only external use of essential oils and always heavily diluted. Why heavily diluted? Well, historically, the British had access to essential oils that were created using solvents or were synthetically created. This led to a distrust of applying these essential oils directly on the skin, without heavy dilution and no ingestion of essential oils. Given the experiences, it is no wonder that a school of thought was born that uses heavy dilution to avoid the problems of synthetic and solvent created essential oils.

The American aromatherapy associations are typically from the British school of thought because their schools teach the British method. The same distrust of essential oil application without heavy dilution has also been passed down, and many aromatherapists will heavily defend what they were taught.

The German method is a school of thought developed in Germany, and focused mainly on aromatic use of essential oils. Little is done with application or ingestion, and may have been due to a low quality of essential oils available to them.

The French method is a school of thought developed in France and focuses on the internal, topical and aromatic use of essential oils. This method advocates the neat application, where essential oils are applied without a carrier oil, and even advocates the ingestion of essential oils because of the distillation method chosen. By using steam distillation, the essential oils produced are high quality, pure, and unadulterated oils. This produced a trust in the quality and effectiveness of essential oils that were safe to use aromatically, topically and internally.

Now when you hear someone talk about essential oils, you will know what school of thought they hail from and what kind of essential oils they are using.

The Toxic Dilemma

This toxic dilemma leads more and more people to want to search out and find new sources for personal care products, makeup, soaps, laundry detergent, dish soap and cleaning supplies in their homes and for their pets.

Most people come to the area of essential oils in order to be able to support their family's health naturally without having to worry about toxic chemicals. I have already talked about synthetics and other toxins and how they negatively affect our health, but why stop at just essential oils? There are so many different areas of our lives that would be benefited by clean and natural products that are toxin-free.

I think it would be best to explore the problem a little further before we search for a solution.

The Toxic Substance Control Act of 1976 by the Environmental Protection Agency (EPA) grandfathered in approximately 62,000 chemicals that were in use at the time without any additional testing. Since that time approximately another 22,000 chemicals have been added into the EPA list and only about 200 of the new chemicals have been tested.

My friend Amanda Uribe, author of *Dig; Unearthing the Leader Within*, had this to say about toxins: "While there are thousands of chemicals in our cleaning products, there are several "favorites" used time and again in the most popular recipes. These "dirty dozen" are the greatest threat to your health and wellness." The "dirty dozen" list is shared later in this chapter.

Let's take a few moments to look at just a few of these chemicals that are part of the 62,000 that were exempted, and key players in the "dirty dozen."

Propylene glycol – An industrial air conditioning and heavy equipment antifreeze, which can be found in laundry detergent and paint. It is known to cause an allergic reaction to the skin and airways and is a developmental and reproductive toxin, but yet it can be found on the ingredient list of many foods and personal care products in the grocery store.

Bisphenol A (BPA) – Originally used as an estrogen supplement before they found out it started causing too many problems. It is a known human carcinogen, is toxic to the brain, heart and other organ system as well as causing developmental and reproductive harm. BPA's use changed over to the hardening of plastics where until 2008 it could be found in baby bottles many other plastics in our homes.

Sodium lauryl sulfate (SLS) – A known allergen to skin and is also known to cause organ system toxicity and developmental and reproductive harm. It is used as the bubbling agent in many soaps, shampoos, and personal care products that are still on the shelves today.

Parabens – A preservative that is a known hormone disruptor and is a carcinogen that causes breast cancer. It is used in approximately 85% of the personal care products on the shelves and also used in many of the foods in the stores.

With products like propylene glycol, BPA, Sodium Lauryl Sulfate and parabens already being listed as part of the 62,000 chemicals that were grandfathered in, how can we know what products on the shelf to use to keep our families healthy?

How safe are your personal care products and cleaning supplies? In 2004, a study done by the Environmental Working Group showed the extent of carcinogens and other toxic chemicals in the products used daily by men and women. The results showed that the average woman uses 12 personal care products, with 168 different chemicals, and the average man uses 6 products, with 85 different chemicals.

This is a pretty scary fact when you consider that, from the time this study was done in 2004, the chemicals in the store-bought personal care products have only increased. In fact the 2015 study by Bionsen, a deodorant maker in London, discovered that the average British woman applies over 515 chemicals daily!

When you consider that Europe has more restrictions on what chemicals are allowed in products, having banned many of the chemicals that are used daily in products the United States, it really is no wonder that cancer rates in United States have skyrocketed.

I'd like to give you a 3 cabinet challenge. Go to your laundry room cabinet, your kitchen sink cabinet, and your bathroom cabinet and compare the ingredients with the following two lists. The first list is a list of carcinogens (cancer causing chemicals) and the second list is a list of other chemicals that are hormone disruptors, allergens or cause harm to your organs, in other words, the "dirty dozen."

List 1 - 94% of women and 69% of men use at least one of these chemicals and 20% of adults are exposed daily to all seven of these top carcinogens.

- 1,4-dioxane
- Acrylamide
- Ethylene Dioxide
- Formaldehyde
- Hydroquinone
- Nitrosamines
- Polycyclic Aromatic Hydrocarbons (PAHs)

List 2 – Here is a list of the "dirty dozen" of chemicals:

- Glycol Esters including propylene glycol
- BPA
- SLS
- Parabens
- Ethanolamines
- Phthalates
- Triclosan

- Sodium Hypochlorite
- Amonia
- Hydroxides
- Petroleum
- Fragrance Chemicals

How did your products do? Would you like to be able to shop for products that are not harmful to you and your family?

It would be nice if we could look towards the same company that we're buying our essential oils from to be able to give us a guarantee on the cleanliness of the products that we need throughout the rest of our house. After all, doesn't it make sense that the essential oil company that has the best dedication to quality, purity, testing and standards would have the same dedication towards any of their other products?

Finding a company that is a trusted source for supplements, fitness and health, personal care products, makeup, soaps, laundry detergent, dish soap and non-toxic cleaning supplies took a lot of stress off my mind. Finding that they are safe for the women, men, children, babies, animals and pets in my home was even better. I found a pure and safe resource for my family to purchase those products from my favorite essential oil company. Would that be a source of comfort to you as well?

Proof In Action – Check The Facts

Let me help you do your own research. Here's a list of questions we've covered so far in this chapter, so call your companies and see what their responses are to these questions.

Grocery Store Oils

- How long have you been in the essential oil business?
- Do you own your own farms?
- Do you test and bottle your own oils?
- Do you use synthetics to avoid being out of stock in a product?
- Do you continually try to improve the quality of your oils?

I Trust The Store Where I Am Buying

- Do you have any obligation to ensure the quality of items on your shelves?
- How do essential oils get on the shelf?
- Do you perform any tests on the essential oils sold in your store?

Science & Testing

- Do you test your essential oils? What tests? How often?
- If an essential oil doesn't meet your standards, what do you do with it?
- Do you resell it? Do you sell it anyway?

- What are your quality standards?
- Do any other companies test your essential oils for quality and purity?
- Are the companies that test your essential oils on your payroll?
- How many essential oil singles and blends do you have?
- Do you have a research team?
- What do they research?
- Do you have any products other than essential oils?

Organic Standards & Regulations

- Does the organic standard apply to essential oils as well?
- Is there really some sort of governing body that monitors the organic standards for essential oils?
- What are the requirements for a section of land before planting seeds?

What School Of Thought?

- What school of thought does your company follow? The British? The Germans? The French?

Part of doing your own research means asking yourself some hard questions too.

The Toxic Problem

- How comfortable are you with the toxins in your home?
- Did you do the 3 cabinet challenge? How did your products fare?

- Would you like to trust your essential oil companies for more products than just essential oils?

While looking at Testing, Standards & Grocery Store Oils, it became apparent that the regulations regarding toxins and chemicals are not very heavily regulated. In the next chapter, I will be looking at the world of Multi-Level Marketing and Network Marketing companies and see what they have to offer in this search for the best essential oil company.

CHAPTER 3

Multi-Level Marketing/Network Marketing

*"Here's my whole marketing idea treat people
the way you want to be treated."*
~Garth Brooks

When talking about Multi-Level Marketing (MLM) companies or network marketing companies, people either love them or hate them with a passion! I have heard many excuses and concerns, but as I investigated more and grew in knowledge about multi-level marketing and network marketing companies the questions seemed to answer themselves, so I decided to list them below and help explain them.

I Don't Want To Do Sales!

One of my first concerns when I heard about MLM companies, was one of being forced to do sales. I certainly don't want to become the pushy salesperson that makes people feel uncomfortable, ruin relationships and have to spend all my time trying to convince people to buy a product they are not interested in anyway. I don't consider myself a salesperson and a job based in sales is not how I wanted to spend my time.

In the past, I had watched my wife join a network marketing company as a candle consultant so that she can get discount prices or free products. She ended up having to buy a bunch of products to have a display, hosted a party and had two friends host a party with their friends and that gave her a little bit of income. This income, however, came from the friends that were eager to come over and obligingly buy a few items as their courteous dues in exchange for the social time, but there was no follow up parties without the work of pushing a friend of a friend to host a party. After all, how many candles, containers, bags, clothes and cooking equipment did people really need?

It is one of these bad experiences that caused people to be jaded towards all MLMs. In reality, it is that specific MLM that they're mad at and distrust. It is their dislike of that one specific pushy sales person that wouldn't take no for an answer, and their fear that if they join they would have to become the same. It is the fear of having to being forced to sell, have inventory, buy monthly and take money from their family's mouths that is holding them hostage. It is important to remember that not all MLMs are the same; there are good MLM companies too.

My favorite essential oil company is a Network Marketing company that doesn't require me to sell to be a part of the company. In fact approximately 90% of the people involved in that company use the products for their own purposes and not for the purpose of sales.

Do I Have To Purchase Monthly?

Having been involved in several Network Marketing companies before, I am always leery of having to make a monthly purchase amount. One company required me to purchase 100 points per month, and instead of being equivalent to about $100, it actually equated to between $150-200 a month.

Yikes, talk about your unexpected costs and feeling like you were handcuffed. We wanted to buy approximately $75/month in products but had to spend more and build up a surplus so that we could cancel our membership for about half the year. This really inefficient system led to a lot of frustration and made us feel trapped.

Now, my wife and I look for companies without a monthly purchase requirement. If they have a requirement, we now have strict requirements; the points better match the dollars, the requirement needs to be only about $50 and I need to be able to cancel at any time, without penalty.

A company that lets me choose if I want to sell, what I want to buy, how much I want to buy, and how often I want to do that is a company that cares about my freedom of choice.

Once again, my favorite essential oil company is a company like that and so much more. Not only do they let me choose if I want to purchase monthly, but if I choose to, the monthly requirement is $50/month, I get points back from my purchases that go up over time, I get free gifts if I stay on the monthly purchase plan, and I can quit whenever I want without penalty.

I'm Paying Inflated Prices!

Cost is the biggest determining factor for most people when making a decision to purchase new products, and essential oils aren't any different. The prevalence of options in the stores and online marketplaces, and the cheapness of many of them, skews people thoughts into thinking that the cheaper oils are better. This means that I hear pretty often that people think they are paying inflated prices with a MLM company, without reference to quality, purity or testing.

Additionally, there is a mistaken thought with a MLM company, that they are somehow paying more just because it is a Network Marketing company, which is charging more money to pay all the people who are part of the compensation plan.

A Network Marketing company is simply selling its products in a different way. Instead of spending a significant portion of the profits of the company to pay advertising to large marketing companies for radio, TV and billboards, and to stores to put their products on the shelves, the Network Marketing company pays advertising money to the families and individuals who are enjoying the products and recommending them to friends.

Another cost comment or excuse is, "I would rather support small businesses than large ones." This implies that the MLM is the large company and the grocery store company is the smaller company. However, the MLM is both a large company AND a small company.

The MLM is Multi-Level Marketing, and each person in that company is considered to have their own business. Their businesses are made up of the single parents, moms, dads, teens, and families stepping out as entrepreneurs and starting their own business. In essence, the MLM is made up of the smallest businesses there is, and supporting them means that you are supporting your neighbor, friend, or family to start and grow their own business and provide for their family.

The next cost objection is the excuse that there are cheaper oils online.

First, you get what you pay for. When you buy cheap things, the quality will also be cheap. You are intentionally choosing the lowest quality when you choose the lowest price. It would be better for you to buy nothing and save, than buy the lowest quality essential oils. As we discussed earlier, the cheapest essential oils are filled with synthetic toxins or are heavily diluted.

Second, when you buy essential oils from an online re-seller, you are trusting the quality of your health to the individual seller. The seller alone is responsible for ensuring the quality of the product, and you are not even guaranteed to get the oil that you bought. The re-sale company is not liable for the quality of the product and is only there to facilitate the sale.

Third, it might never arrive, and worse still it could arrive and be a bottle that was emptied, and re-filled with toilet water. Unless you buy your oils directly from the manufacturer, you have no guarantee of quality.

The last portion to the cost objection I've had about multi-level marketing companies is a complaint that the oils are the same quality is what you find in the grocery store. This is usually a secondary complaint to cost or to higher prices that we've already addressed in the past 2 chapters.

We've already covered how quality essential oils can differ even in the grocery store depending on if they are diluted, extracted using solvents, or just plain being done just for smell. Quality isn't determined by selling in a store. Quality is determined by the standards, policies, procedures, testing and purity of the company that sells them.

What I've noticed is that the complaint really isn't based on whether or not the oils are better or the same quality in the grocery store, but they're already using a particular brand from the grocery store and are justifying to themselves why they shouldn't switch.

I find by asking them where they currently get the oils or what brand they use reaffirms my suspicion and I offer to share with them essential oils from my favorite company. At any rate, when I share with someone products from my favorite essential oil company, they recognize the difference in quality, purity, and strength. The previous complaints that the oils are the same quality store is no longer valid because once you experience a higher-quality essential oil, there's no reason to purchase from anywhere else.

My favorite essential oil company does whatever it can to reduce the production costs of its products, and passes on that reduction to its members. One such way is on one of their farms where they produce an abundance of high quality, earthquake resistant bricks which are sold inexpsively to the local populace. When the proceeds are used to reduce the cost of running the farm and the distilling of essential oils, the cost savings is passed onto you.

Ask Yourself...

Is quality worth paying for? Do you like helping small businesses, and friends? Would you like a friend who cares about you to help you figure out how to use essential oils and answer your questions? Would you prefer to get a product with a quality guarantee?

Isn't It Just A Pyramid Scheme?

Another objection that I have heard someone say is "Oh, it is a network marketing company, how do I know it's not just a pyramid scheme?" Well here's the answer; a pyramid scheme or a Ponzi scheme, as it's otherwise known, is where only an exchange of money is occurring but not any products or services. An exchange of products or services is the key to distinguishing between if it's a Ponzi scheme or a legitimate business. Besides that, Ponzi schemes are illegal. How long would network marketing and MLM companies last if they were performing illegal activities?

I have been told, "The organization structure of a network marketing company has to be a pyramid scheme because it looks like a pyramid!" It is humorous to think the key word is pyramid and not scheme! Look at your job, the company you work for, what is the organizational structure of that company look like? I'm betting you have one CEO, a few high-level managers, a greater number of lower- level managers and finally all the rest of the employees. The organizational structure looks like what shape? A pyramid! Oh no, it must be a pyramid scheme!

Well, that's ridiculous. If we were to look at the structure of any organization most likely it also looks like a pyramid. Just look at your church, a non-profit or even a volunteer event: you have the leader, the managers, and everyone else. That forms another pyramid, so obviously the key word is not pyramid but scheme.

When Bernie Madoff received money from people, he promised them huge rates of return on their investments. In actuality, he only sent them a small portion of their money back and pocketed the rest. When he did not perform the investment services he promised, that is when it became a Ponzi scheme.

I remember when I was a teenager, I got a letter in the mail from a classmate that said, "This system is so excellent, I will make you much more money than you will be spending. Simply send a dollar to the 10 names on this list, then retype the list removing the top name and adding your name to the bottom and send out to 10 friends." It was so tempting at the time, the promises of quick, easy money, and all I had to do was spend less than $15 and I could make millions, just like the testimonials in the letter said.

Thankfully I recognized it for what it was, but first, even as I was reading it, my brain was scheming and looking for loopholes. I was tempted to not send $1 to the 10 names above and instead just send it to 10 friends. I realized immediately that was wrong, and since I was tempted to do so, everyone else on that list that I sent it to would be tempted also.

Additionally, this guarantee of millions, the letter so faithfully talked about and gave testimonials for, really couldn't be true. As I analyzed the letter even more I questioned it more. How can they have testimonials in this letter if it's always sent on to the next person before the results come back to the first person? I didn't know it then, but that was a pyramid scheme, and illegal; there were no products of services being exchanged.

As years passed, we've moved into the digital age and I have seen multiple emails come across my screen promising me rewards, gift cards, money and even huge donations to wonderful causes if I would just copy and send the message on to all of my contacts. That earlier letter that I had received helped me to recognize all the rest of these schemes for what they were.

Now these messages are just labeled as spam and deleted, but how many people have fallen prey to them, have sent money or even sent it on? All they really do is give you a whole bunch of empty promises without results. That is what a pyramid scheme or a Ponzi scheme does; it gives you promises with small amounts of money in return for huge amounts of money on your part with no real products or services changing place.

Looking strictly at the definition, the US Social Security system is the biggest legal Ponzi scheme, because it promises rewards that are only monetarily based and has no products or services exchanging hands. While I have been paying into the social security system for decades, I fully expect that the entire system will be totally bankrupt by the time I would be drawing anything from that system.

I don't like pyramid schemes, and I refuse to voluntarily be part of them.

When I pay a tax advising and accounting company, they advise me on how to do my taxes and submit my taxes. When I call a lawyer, they provide legal services. When I call a plumber, they come and fix the problem. This by nature makes these companies not pyramid schemes because they actually provide a product or service.

But what about network marketing companies, why are they not pyramid schemes? Because they provide products and services! An MLM or network marketing company provides you with products when you pay them money. You are not sending them money and getting nothing but promises in return. Instead what you have is an exchange of goods and services, just as if you went into an actual physical grocery store and bought bananas or to an amusement park to ride roller coasters.

Well, ok, but what about the commissions their distributors receive, isn't that a pyramid scheme? No, they provided multiple services: advertising for the company, they gave you information about a product and showed you how to order it, and hopefully even educated you on how to use it! Shouldn't they get paid for providing a service too?

Ask Yourself...

What product or service does this company produce? Is there only money exchanging hands?

I Don't Want To Keep Product On Hand!

In my opinion, the worst negative I've heard about network marketing companies is sometimes people have to buy huge amounts of product to have on hand to sell. I've heard of people having to spend $1,000 to $10,000 or more on having product on hand so that when people want to buy something they can sell it to them right then.

In this case the only one making any money at all is the company itself. The company gets their money up front and the person taking the risk is the distributor or reseller on the promise that they will be able to resell it. This saddens me. How many people do you know who have bags, leggings, socks, lipsticks, soaps, candles and more filling their closet, car or garage and are hoping to sell them all off?

If a product is truly exceptional, you wouldn't need people to pay you to keep a huge inventory on hand. The company wouldn't need the individual distributors to hold all the risk of future sales, but instead would be willing to hold the risk themselves.

Additionally, as the individual is keeping the product for resale and it spoils or the packaging is damaged and still sold, doesn't that make the company look bad as a whole? Surely distributors will come up with creative ways of discounting products and getting them off their shelves, and recouping some of their losses. Wouldn't it be better if the company were so sure of the quality of its product that it's willing to hold all of its products in its warehouse to wait for orders and even to reship something that's damaged, spoiled or lost in shipping? My favorite essential oil company is like this; it holds all the product itself and even reships damaged, spoiled or lost shipments.

A truly exceptional company would have such a quality product that it would be willing to shoulder the risk itself. It would have the integrity that it would not require distributors to keep an inventory of products on hand and instead would ship the products on-demand. It would be willing to let the quality of the products stand for itself, not demand huge buy-in amounts from new distributors and instead provide a way for their distributors to share products at a low buy-in amount. The customers, after recognizing the quality, would come to the company saying, "We want this product and we're going to wait for it to show up."

My favorite essential oil company is a company with a very low buy-in amount, doesn't require me to have huge amounts of products on hand, and enables every person that buys product to become a distributor if they choose. In fact, when I first bought products for myself I already had everything I needed to be a distributor if I chose to become one.

Would you like a company that made it easy for you to start a home business?

You Have To Get In From The Start To Make Money!

The last problem that people have with network marketing companies crosses the boundary of whether we're talking about essential oils or any other network marketing company, and that is the belief that you have to get in from the start of the company to make any money.

As far as I'm concerned there are three factors that determine whether or not that is true, the Five-Year rule, the quality of the products, and the compensation plan.

The first factor, the Five-Year rule, is determined by the age of the company. With start up businesses the first five years are the most volatile, and many do not survive. This is also true with network marketing companies, after they have passed the 5-year mark, then they have a greater chance of surviving. However, if you had joined that company in the first 5 years, you would have been in more danger of losing everything than in succeeding big. The company was still figuring out how to survive and was developing its policies, procedures, and standards for quality.

The second factor, quality of the products, determines how much demand there is going to be for that company's products. If the quality is poor, then no matter how cheap the products are, the company simply will not last and you will not make any money in that company. The second biggest rule in network marketing is that you must have a product that you can stand behind, because you have to be a product of the product. Your friends, neighbors, enemies and potential customers are watching you to see what products you use, to see if this is a fad. They are watching to see if there's anything in what you are saying that is true or untrue. If you aren't a product of the product people see right through you. The easiest way to be a product to the product is to fully and completely believe in the product that you are selling.

You can believe in a good product, believe in a great product, but you can't believe in a horrible product! You might be able to fool all the people some of the time, some of the people all of the time, but not all the people all the time. If your product is a fraud it will be known quickly, and you will never make any money.

If, however, your product is a truly exceptional product where the quality stands for itself, and someone will experience the difference by trying it, then your product will convince them better than any of your words. Your product will create a paradigm shift from everything else they knew before, and there is nothing to stop you from growing and making money in that business.

The third factor, the compensation plan, is the single biggest factor that can determine whether or not you will make any money in a company or not. If the compensation plan is set up so that the company is stingy with their profit sharing, the competition is cut- throat with your downline and other members, and it is too hard to go from one level to the next, then a business in that company is doomed from the beginning.

I've heard of multiple network marketing companies where it hurts you to teach your downline how to sell efficiently because if your downline outranks you they can be removed from your organization, and if you make too much money you can be kicked out of the company!

If the company, however, is smart with their business plan, and pays their distributors well, then the distributors will work hard to keep ranking up and earning money because the reward is worth it. A company that treats its employees well will keep its employees, and a network marketing company that is treating its distributors well will keep the distributors.

Teamwork is the easiest way to grow, and a network marketing company that supports teamwork and generously pays people for their efforts is one company where there will be people making lots of money!

Ask Yourself...
Would you like to work with a company that makes it easy for you to grow? Would you like to work with a team that you will never lose?

Proof In Action – Check The Facts

After reading about the most common questions and objections to Network Marketing and MLM companies, I'm sure it gave you things to think about. Here are a few questions to ask any Network Marketing or MLM company and yourself too.

I Don't Want To Do Sales!

- Am I required to sell your product?

Do I Have To Purchase Monthly?

- If I join your company, am I required to make a monthly purchase?
- Are product points equal to dollars?

I'm Paying Inflated Prices!

- Is quality worth paying for?
- Do you like helping small businesses, and friends?
- Would you like a friend who cares about you to help you figure out how to use essential oils and answer your questions?
- Would you prefer to get a product with a quality guarantee?

Isn't It Just A Pyramid Scheme?

- What product or service does this company produce?
- Is there only money exchanging hands?

I Don't Want To Keep Product On Hand!

- Would you like a company that made it easy for you to start a home business?
- Does your company require me to have inventory on hand to sell?
- How much do I have to buy to become a new distributor?
- Do you reship products missing or lost in shipment?

You Have To Get In From The Start To Make Money!

- Does your company make it easy for me to grow?
- Do I ever lose downline members if they outrank me?

While there are surely some network marketing and MLM companies that trick people, have unreasonable rules and shady business practices, it is not true for all of them. In the next chapter, you will see what my favorite Essential Oil Company is and how it measures up.

CHAPTER 4

The Best Essential Oil Company!

*"If you want to be the best, you have to do things that
other people aren't willing to do."*
~Michael Phelps

Young Living Essential Oils

What makes Young Living the best essential oil company?
Here is what makes up the Young Living Difference!

- Seed to Seal® Quality Commitment
- 25 Years of Industry Leadership
- 21 Corporate and Partner Farms – And Growing
- 600+ Life Changing Products
- Over 270 Single Essential Oils & Blends
- Savvy Minerals Makeup
- Thieves® Non-Toxic Cleaning
- Supplements, Fitness & Health
- Personal Care Products
- Weight Management
- Men's Health
- Kids & Babies
- Animals & Pets

- 50+ Highly Trained Scientists
- 2 State-of –the-Art Corporate Quality Labs
- 12+ Independent Partner Labs
- Started D. Gary Young, Young Living Foundation
- Pays 100% of the Administrative Costs
- 100% of Donations Provide Direct Impact
- 250,000+ Individual Lives Impacted
- 170 Causes & Charities Supported
- 32 International Markets
- 26 Offices and Experience Centers Worldwide
- The Original Essential Oil Network Marketing Company
- Over 6 million Members
- 3,300+ Global Employees
- Exceeding $1.5 Billion in Revenue Annually Since 2015

I'll give you four main reasons below, and explain them and others from above in greater detail in the following chapters.

First, D. Gary Young's passion for learning as much as he could about essential oils transferred into his desire to produce the purest quality essential oils in the world, and his heartfelt desire to care for people was infused into Young Living's culture and company from the start. These factors permeate every part of Young Living's culture and legacy making it more like a family than a business, caring more about people than profit, and taking the stewardship of our planet seriously. The industry-leading Seed to Seal® commitment brings you the purest essential oils and infused products on Earth through conscious sourcing, science, and standards.

Second, the quality and purity of Young Living's products is unequaled in the essential oil industry and has been perfected over the 25 years they've been in business. The quality of the product speaks for itself. I don't have to convince you that Young Living is better; I just need to hand you a sample of Young Living Essential Oils and let you experience the power, strength, and effectiveness for yourself.

Third, the distinctive qualities of Young Living are Gary's education and training, the Seed to Seal® guarantee, owning their own farms, the distillation method, the testing they do on their products, the research and development, and the dedication to a toxin-free lifestyle.

The last factor is Young Living's mission to foster a community of healing and discovery and their dedication to help people find wellness, purpose, and abundance in their lives. Their commitment to sharing wellness, purpose and abundance can be seen by following how the money flows through Young Living. First, it is apparent how Young Living abundantly supports the D. Gary Young, Young Living Foundation. Second, Young Living's members receive benefits and free gifts for shopping in their own store. Third, the choice of a Network Marketing structure means that the money that would be spent on advertising is instead given back to its members rather than other companies. Helping people find wellness, purpose and abundance is what Young Living is all about.

In the next few chapters I'll be going into detail on all of these points and so much more. If you doubt what I'm saying in any of these sections, you are welcome to research the information yourself, but in the end I believe you will come to the same conclusion: Young Living is the best essential oil company.

Why It Is My Favorite Essential Oil Company

Young Living Essential Oils is my favorite essential oil company for many reasons, but the first one is as follows. My wife and I were looking for something, anything, that would support our daughter Jubilee's health when she was hospitalized for a month at 8 months old. Young Living Essential Oils supported her health when nothing else could. I would love to give you more of a description on this, but I'm not allowed to because that would make it commercial speech according to the FDA.

After finding something to support Jubilee's health, we focused on figuring out if we had the best essential oil company, as well as what else could they could do for us. We wanted to know what company had the highest quality, purity, and standards. Very soon transparency, following the money and motives, who owns the farms, and science and testing became important too.

We figured out that two of the most important determining factors for a company were the amount of time they had in service and the amount of training that they had in producing high-quality essential oils.

At the time we started, Young Living had been around for almost 20 years (now 25 years), and its founder Gary Young had been studying essential oils for an additional 10 years before he started his company. No other essential oil company came close to any of those numbers. Several essential oil companies started between 2006-2013 after seeing the opportunity in the marketplace and many more companies started up after Young Living experienced massive growth in 2013 and 2014.

My research showed that companies that had been exclusively focused on product areas like cleaning supplies and vitamins suddenly had essential oil lines, and companies have sprung up out of nowhere with essential oils. Both of these types of essential oil newcomers have also claimed they have the highest quality essential oils, with no experience, supply or infrastructure.

Furthermore, Gary Young had figured out how to produce high-quality essential oils that were so much more potent than anything else on the marketplace that he started calling them therapeutic grade. The funny thing is that, in the next few years, every new and existing essential oil company suddenly had "therapeutic grade essential oils."

Since there is no regulating agency for the quality and purity of essential oils, the new companies could make whatever claims they wanted. But I ask you, which one most likely has the better quality, the true therapeutic grade, the company who had 10 years of research and experience, or the companies that saw a new descriptive term, and decided that they wanted to use it too?

I found that not one other company had all the factors. They were failing in one or more of these areas, so not one was using the purest method distillation, had their own farms, were totally transparent allowing you to visit and tour, tested their oil inside their company and with third party companies, and basically monitored where the seeds went in the ground all the way though cultivation, distillation, testing and bottling.

What this means is that Young Living is the only company that is not a broker of essential oils, meaning that they know for sure the quality of their entire process from start to finish. They do not have to take somebody else's word for it at some point in the process. Young Living, contrary to the other companies, is not just getting a shipment in, relabeling as their own and sending it back out again like a broker, but rather is growing, monitoring, and verifying the process.

Young Living monitors:

- What seeds to plant.
- In what type of ground their seeds are being planted.
- How their plants are taken care of and what is sprayed on them.
- How the plants are harvested.
- What conditions are used in their distillation.
- If the essential oils meet their rigorous quality and testing standards.
- How the blends are mixed.
- How the oils are bottled.
- And so much more!

Learning all that about Young Living was exciting, and no one else even came close! On top of all that, we found out that Young Living had taken their dedication to quality, toxin-free products and had developed products for every area of our lives that were toxin-free, safe, and effective.

Young Living has vitamins and supplements, personal care products, mineral-based makeup, cleaning supplies and household products, and products for weight management, men, women, kids, babies, animals and pets, fitness and health, and even cookware. I will go over these things in more detail in chapter 9.

Gary's Story

The world of essential oils in one way or another revolves around Young Living Essential Oils and its founder, D. Gary

Young. As I said in chapter 2, when everybody else tries to claim that they're better than one company, it really does point to that one company as the true leader in the industry.

Young Living Essential Oils owes their unparalleled quality, unmatched purity, and unrivaled testing and standards to D. Gary Young, an unmatched authority on essential oils.

Throughout his life, D. Gary Young:

- Authored and co-authored 21 different research papers
- Authored 12 books on essential oils,
- Substantially contributed to 8 editions of essential oil desk references, pocket references and an animal desk reference with his research, lectures, seminars, workshops, experiences and scientific publications that were compiled with other expert practitioners and physicians in the use of therapeutic essential oils.

When Gary first got interested in essential oils he went to study from the experts worldwide 10 years before even starting Young Living as a company. He studied from a recognized expert in essential oils, Jean-Claude Lapraz, in 1985 in Geneva Switzerland, and in Paris with Paul Belaiche, MD and Daniel Pénoël, a recognized expert and co-author of a French book on aromatherapy, called "l'aromathérapie exactement" or loosely translated as "Exact Aromatherapy."

Gary's final studies before beginning Young Living involved working directly with a French Lavender grower and distiller, Jean-Noel Landel, in Provence France. It was there he was introduced to and studied directly under the renowned distillation and essential oil quality expert Henri Viaud. Mr. Viaud is the author of the book on the quality considerations for steam distilled essential oils called, "Huiles Essentielles - Hydrolats" or loosely translated as "Essential Oils By Steam Distillation." Mr. Viaud only had one student, Gary Young, who he taught all of his expertise in distillation. Later, Mr. Viaud recognized D. Gary Young as the new master in the art of distillation.

After starting Young Living, Gary continued to study with experts on essential oils at Cairo University, Egypt and Andalou University in Eskisehir, Turkey.

Additionally, to further his knowledge on gas chromatography, Gary studied both at the Albert Vielle Laboratory in Grasse, France and with the world's foremost authority in chromatography, Herve Casabianca, Phd. Later, Dr. Cassabianca traveled to the US and Ecuador to train the finer points of gas chromatography/ mass spectrometry to the scientific staff at Young Living.

Furthermore, Gary Young has personally trained over 50 scientists at Young Living in both the realm of quality, standards and testing, and the distillation, blending and purity of essential oils.

People were so important to Gary that he constantly pushed himself as well, rarely resting because the people needed him, and they needed the products, farms and distilleries.

I've heard many stories where people told Gary that a plan or innovation or design of his would never work, but time and time again he would prove them all wrong. Gary started a living legacy, by bringing therapeutic grade essential oils to the United States and the rest of the world, by the numerous lives that are changed daily because of his work, and by creating a company so dedicated to quality, standards and purity that its mission and direction would last even after his death.

With credentials such as these, how can any other company claim that they are the world's authority in essential oils?

Distillation Methods

One of the most expensive forms of distillation today is steam distillation. It also happens to be the purest and cleanest method, which is why Young Living made the decision to build steam distillation facility at each of its farms.

With Young Living, over 90% of the 120 different single essential oils that are extracted use the steam distillation method. Other methods include hydro-distillation, cold pressing citrus oils from the rind, and since there is no other way, the use of food grade grain alcohol is used to extract the essential oils of Jasmine and Neroli. But, even still, because of cost, most essential companies will not use steam distillation for the cheapest essential oils like Lemongrass and Cedarwood, or the most expensive oils like Rose.

Using steam distillation to distill Rose essential oil is the most expensive method, but it shows a lot about the company and their dedication to quality. Using steam distillation, it takes about 2,000 pounds of rose petals to make about one gallon of Rose essential oil. To put it in perspective, that is equivalent to using 50 pounds of rose petals for each 5 ml bottle.

As you can imagine, this is a really expensive method to use, but quality is worth the price, and a bottle of Rose essential oil created using this method costs about $190. Can you see why in an earlier chapter, I said run from a company that charges $10 for their giant size bottle of Rose essential oil?

In December 2016, I had the opportunity to help with the Idaho Balsam Fir harvest at the Highland Flats farm in Northern Idaho. What a thrilling and eye-opening experience as I participated in every area of harvesting and distillation.

When I first arrived, I found out that Young Living had a wonderful relationship with all of the landowners in the area. About four decades ago there was a Christmas tree farm spanning from Eastern Washington through Idaho to Montana, but after the owner's death, the children sold the farm to farmers and other landowners.

This meant if the farmers wanted to utilize the land for farming, ranching, or housing, they had to pay $500 dollars an hour for someone to cut down the trees and burn them. But Gary Young, the founder of Young Living Essential Oils, had managed to make a better arrangement with the farmers. He would provide, free of charge, equipment to cut down and chip the wild grown trees in the winter according to the farmer's specifications. Later, in the springtime, he would come back to remove the stumps and return the land to useable form for farming, also for free.

My first day in the field started off with a ride in the semi trailer with Gary Young and two other distributors. The semi-truck is where all of the wood chips would be put as trees were cut, and chipped for distillation. As Gary drove to the farm, the distributors and I engaged him in conversation, and you could tell that he enjoyed every moment of what he did, was a wealth of information, and his dedication to his work was tremendous!

What impressed me most was that Gary had a team of people out working the fields and yet he still came out to work the harvest and spend time with distributors. His dedication was so great that, even though he'd hurt himself riding his snowmobile with his son the week before, he was still working through the pain without complaint to be a part of that harvest. I soon learned that dedication was typical Gary, to work through pain because he cared so much about all of us.

The most exciting moment for me in the semi truck was when Gary pulled over when we were at the last few turns on the way to the farm, and turned to me and said "All right, go ahead and drive." It was a dream come true. I got to drive the 60 foot semi-trailer down the road and through a 90-degree turn in the snow. I didn't screw up, and I even got a compliment. I then pulled over, and the other two distributors took turns making their own turns. What a thrilling adventure!

The adventure didn't end there. I drove a skid steer and cut trees myself, drove the team of draft horses to drag the log to the collection point, and threw smaller trees and branches into the chipper- shredder!

At one point, I got to sit with Gary in the feller-buncher and watch as he harvested tree after tree. What an artist he was, so skilled in cutting trees and faster than everyone else! He was tireless, and worked harder and longer than anybody else in that field. In fact, when our group was done working in the field for the day, Gary stayed and worked another 8 hours!

Back at the distillery, the room smelled amazing as we worked and watched the essential oils being distilled from the wood chips. We helped unload wood chips from the back of the semi trailers, drove skid steers to dump loads of chipped Idaho Balsam Fir into the still, and stomped down the wood chips in the still.

The still is about 8 feet around and 20 feet tall, and is filled bucket load by bucket load, while people stomp down the material in the still. When full, we helped put the cone-shaped lid on and watched the steam distillation procedure begin. We learned that Gary's desire to produce the best quality essential oils had required him to climb into a still and watch as the steam left the chamber.

His resulting analysis led to the redesign of the dome-shaped lid into a cone-shaped lid, because it produces a higher grade of essential oil. The cone-shaped lid allows the steam to leave immediately instead of having to curl around a few times until it finds the opening.

Hours later, we watched as the Idaho Balsam Fir essential oil arrived in the separator and naturally divided itself into oil and water. The essential oil is taken off the top and filtered through a coffee filter to remove any debris.

A sample is collected from each batch of essential oil, and tested for quality, purity, and therapeutic properties before being ready to be put into stainless steel drums. The stainless steel drums are sealed with tamper resistant locking strips for transport by Young Living trucks to the Young Living bottling facility. Even though the essential oils never leave Young Living's control, the security measures are in place to ensure that nothing tampers with the pure, therapeutic grade quality. Each drum is tested again when it arrives at the Young Living bottling facility to verify the quality.

As an added bonus to just being able to experience the entire process and help out, we each received a 5ml bottle of

Idaho Balsam Fir, which we filled ourselves from the batch we helped make.

The testing facilities are on-site, and we were given a full tour and demonstration of the testing procedures. The machines have to be cleaned between every test, and multiple tests are run per day. Essential oils that do not meet Young Living's strict standards are not used or resold; they are discarded.

When the distillation process is over, the woodchips are hoisted out, put in a dump truck and dumped in the field to cool. In the spring the mountain of woodchips are freely given to a local nursery, which mixes them with soil and sells the mulch for profit.

What an incredible relationship Young Living has with the local landowners and an unbeatable dedication to quality.

In addition to this, Young Living has begun growing their own trees on their own land. Every year they plant another batch of seedlings to ensure a renewable resource for the future. Since it takes between 10-15 years to grow a tree to maturity, it is a big undertaking to properly forecast future demand, but this is part of Young Living's commitment to quality.

Would you like to work with an essential oil company with that dedication to quality?

Own Farms & Partner Farms

Gary was once told by one of his mentors, "The time will come, if you don't grow it, you won't have it to distill!" Gary took that to heart, and that's why Young Living currently has 8 of their own farms with on-site distillation facilities and staff working on and monitoring the process of the plants as they go through different stages of development, all the way through the point of distillation, testing and prepping for shipment.

Young Living also has 13 partner farms, which are thoroughly vetted through all processes and procedures to make sure that they are coinciding with the Seed to Seal® standards and policies of Young Living. These farms are given zero tolerance of breaking the rules, and any farm that breaks the rules loses its right to work with Young Living again.

Young Living Farms are also transparent; they encourage you to go and check out their farms, take a tour of their distilleries, and see the quality for yourself.

My family has done this.

We have visited 4 farms and a partner farm and have even just stopped by the farm in St. Maries, Idaho and asked if we could have a tour. Even though they were distilling a very important essential oil at that time, the distillery manager gave us a tour of the entire distillery.

He took his time to explain every part of the distillation and testing process, answered numerous questions and showed us what was behind every single door. At the end of the tour, the distillery manager asked us if we had any questions and my wife turned and asked what was behind one last door. He immediately reached out and opened the door to reveal the janitor's closet!

Talk about transparency; that tour was given and finished even before they found out we were Young Living members!

Wouldn't it be nice to work with an essential oil company that believes in transparency?

Seed to Seal® & A Dedication To Quality

Almost 25 years ago Gary Young established the Seed to Seal® quality system, which makes Young Living stand out as the most unique essential oil company, let alone network marketing company in the world. Gary knew that quality was so important that he made a commitment to quality a standard early on, and constantly pushed the envelope to get more and more quality in every single product he produced. He was constantly designing, testing, and innovating.

Seed to Seal® started off as a 5 part process that went from **1-SEED**, **2-CULTIVATE**, **3-DISTILL**, **4-TEST**, and **5-SEAL**; a start to finish quality commitment for everything from where the seeds go in the ground to when the lid goes on the bottle.

During the **SEED** phase, Young Living ensured things such as the type of land that was to be used, verifying that it had been pesticide- free for 50 years, and the types of seeds that were put into the soil. For lavender for instance, they use the seeds from the biggest, bushiest, most fragrant lavender plants in the field as the seeds for the next year's crops.

During the **CULTIVATION** phase, no pesticides or herbicides are sprayed on the plants. Only workers, who love their job, are allowed to work with the plants and they hand-weed between the plants and hoe between the rows. Additionally, they use only natural fertilizers like worm casing fertilizer, plant matter left over from distillation and even floral water sprayed on the plants, because Young Living knows that whatever is on your plants and in your soil is what goes into your oils. Lastly, as harvest time approaches, Young Living tests their plants in the field to make sure that they are ready for harvest, ensuring that they get the maximum amount of therapeutic properties in your essential oils.

During the **DISTILL** phase, Young Living uses steam distillation and documents the data necessary to produce the highest quality oils, including volume of plant material, curing time needed, steam temperature, distillation time, and any special procedures for that type of oil.

During the **TEST** phase, Young Living performs 21 different tests in triplicate, two different times, and verifies there is nothing in those essential oils that doesn't belong there. This rigorous battery of tests is performed to make certain that your essential oils are free from any synthetics, adulterants or chemicals.

During the **SEAL** phase, the blends are mixed and the singles and blends are bottled, each batch is tested again, and then the labels are put on the bottles before they are ready to be shipped out.

The five phases of Seed to Seal® were continually improved upon as well, so now those five phases become part of the three pillars of the Seed to Seal® quality guarantee, which are **SOURCING, SCIENCE,** and **STANDARDS**.

The **SOURCING** pillar includes the seed and cultivation phases, but also includes the partnership principles and dedication towards sustainable, conscientious sourcing with priority on quality, sensitivity to community impact, and mindfulness towards conserving ecosystems.

The **SCIENCE** pillar includes the last part of the cultivation phase, and adds to it the distillation and testing phases. All of the testing and quality assurance portions of Young Living fit within this Science pillar. Young Living has more than 50 highly trained scientists using 2 state- of-the-art labs to test product samples internally, and uses multiple independent, respected and accredited labs around the world to ensure that the high quality standards are met throughout the entire process. Finally, this pillar includes all of the research and development done within Young Living to include creating formulas and new items to provide families with essential oil infused products that are safe, clean and effective.

The **STANDARDS** pillar includes the seal phase, and also encompasses the rest of the process. At this phase, Young Living creates its standards and policies to ensure that they are being a good steward of natural resources, and creates the agreements for ethical and sustainable sourcing of rare botanicals, uplifting local communities, and identifying new partners to source pure essential oils and ingredients, ethically and legally.

Ask Yourself...

Does your essential oil company perform 21 different tests in triplicate, two different times, to verify your essential oils are free of synthetics, adulterants, and chemicals and contain the highest amount of therapeutic properties? Does your essential oil company use inside and respected independent laboratories to test your essential oils?

The Solution For Toxin-Free Living

The solution to toxin-free living is actually quite simple; it involves a concept I want to introduce you to called transfer-buying. Transfer-buying happens after you recognize the sheer number of toxins throughout your home and you want to stop buying the bad products and instead start buying products that support your health. But figuring out how to change the location where you're purchasing cleaning products, supplements, personal care products and other things throughout your house isn't always easy. Who do you trust now?

My family decided to use Young Living products everywhere in our house, to live a toxin-free lifestyle. Going through the research time to determine which essential oil company has the best dedication to quality, purity, testing and standards gave me a great trust in Young Living. They have the same quality guarantee on their vitamins, supplements, cleaning products, and personal care products that we need throughout the rest of our house.

On top of that, the research showed me what the truth was about the Toxic Dilemma, and showed me the need to live a toxin-free lifestyle.

My family now uses nothing but Young Living personal care products, makeup and cleaning supplies, because we know that what we have is quality products that are free of synthetics, chemicals, toxins, and fillers. Finding a company that I trust to transfer the purchases that I was making in my home was something that took a lot of stress off my mind.

The great thing about transfer-buying is that I do not need to spend any more money. I don't need to add money to my budget or make it work somehow to buy Young Living products, I simply transfer the money I was spending on cleaning supplies, personal care product, and makeup. The products are toxin-free, safe and effective.

Additionally, many of the products, like the Thieves® Household Cleaner, come in a really concentrated form, so we end up saving money by getting about 30 bottles of cleaner out of the same bottle. It also replaced our need to buy every other cleaner in our house, saving even more money.

Proof In Action – Check The Facts

Here is the list of items we've covered so far in this chapter. Feel free to call Young Living customer care at 1-800-371-3515 and see what they say about themselves in each of these areas.

Young Living Essential Oils

- The Seed to Seal® Quality Commitment.
- Young Living been in business for more than 25 years..
- Have currently 8 corporate farms and 13 partner farms.
- Sell more than 600+ Life Changing Products
- Over 270 Single Essential Oils & Blends

Why It Is My Favorite Essential Oil Company

Young Living Monitors:
- What seeds to plant.
- How their plants are taken care and what is sprayed on them.
- How the plants are harvested.
- What conditions are used for each variety of botanical in distillation.
- How the blends are mixed.
- How the oils are bottled.
- If the essential oils meet their rigorous quality and testing standards.

Gary's Story

- Gary worked on every farm and was constantly designing, testing, and innovating.
- Gary studied with masters of distillation and testing throughout the world, including in Switzerland, France, Egypt, and Turkey.

Distillation Methods

- Over 90% of the 120 different single essential oils that are extracted are done through the use of steam distillation.
- Other methods include:
- Hydro-distillation for resins.
- Cold pressing citrus oils from the rind.
- Food grade grain alcohol is used to extract the essential oils of Jasmine and Neroli.

Seed to Seal® & A Dedication To Quality

- Young Living scientists perform 21 different tests in triplicate, two different times, to verify your essential oils are free of synthetics, adulterants, and chemicals and contain the highest amount of therapeutic properties.
- Uses 2 state-of-the-art labs to test product samples internally and multiple independent, respected and accredited labs around the world to ensure that the high quality standards are met throughout the entire process.
- Gary Young personally trained over 50 scientists at Young Living in both the realm of quality, standards and testing, and the distillation, blending and purity of essential oils.

The Solution For Toxin-Free Living

- Using transfer-buying to replace toxic products in your house with safe alternatives.
- Saving money while transfer-buying and concentrated Young Living products.

Now that we have found the best essential oil company, Young Living Essential Oils, feel free to check the facts yourself and get your own answers. In the next chapter I will be discussing further the testing and standards of Young Living and their research and development!

CHAPTER 5

Testing and Standards

"I do have impossibly high standards."
~Kate Winslet

No Compromising

First and foremost, everything I learned about Young Living impressed me greatly! At the heart of Young Living is the desire to never compromise on quality and purity. In fact one of the first things I learned was that Young Living would rather go without an essential oil than compromise on quality.

Melissa Essential Oil is an extremely expensive oil to produce, and if it is done right the cost is about $165 per 5 ml bottle. After a batch of this expensive oil was produced, the testing revealed that this particular batch didn't meet Young Living standards, so Gary Young poured it out on the floor, rather than resell it. Because he loved people so much, he didn't want to give them an inferior product!

Additionally, years later, when there was a worldwide shortage on Helichrysum Essential Oil, a supplier that wanted to become one of their partner farms came to Young Living and said they had a huge batch of Helichrysum Essential Oil. But when Gary smelled that Helichrysum, he recognized there was something wrong with that batch of essential oil, because he was one of less than a dozen people in the world that could detect deficiencies in an essential oil by smelling it. This was his first warning that something was wrong with the essential oil.

After running it through Young Living's thorough testing, they found out that the Helichrysum had been augmented with a synthetic. The batch of oil was quickly refused and the supplier blacklisted.

While Young Living is a company that will not compromise on quality no matter how much profit is involved, it is sad to note that shortly thereafter, one of the competitors suddenly had a supply of Helichrysum to sell.

Would you like to be a part of a company that would rather go without an essential oil than compromise on quality?

Testing Before Harvesting & Distillation

In the weeks and days before harvest, Young Living scientists perform a Brix Test, which measures of the amount of solid matter in a liquid sample to get an idea of the health of the plant. The Brix rating they receive is compared to the historical Brix ratings recorded for that plant as it nears harvest and distillation, and when the numbers match they know they're ready to harvest.

Variations in the growing season, such as low temperatures, heavy rains, high temperatures or little rain, will greatly affect the time for harvest. Daily Brix level testing is performed, as it nears harvest time for that plant, to determine the glucose content, which helps determine the optimal day and time of day for harvest.

A small amount of the plant is cut and run through a test distill, and sent for gas chromatography/mass spectrometer (GC/MS) testing to determine the chemical profile, which identifies the therapeutic properties for that essential oil.

Sometimes, a few sample distills are performed to determine when new plant types are ready to be harvested and to see if that particular plant has enough benefits to merit further cultivation.

While at the Idaho Balsam Fir harvest, I participated in gathering samples and preparations for test distills being performed on Western Red Cedar and got a chance to sample the oil that was produced. It smelled amazing!

Types & Number Of Tests

Beside the Brix test that is run before harvest, Young Living also performs 21 different tests on their essential oils to ensure that their members receive the highest quality essential oils in the world. Not only do they perform 21 separate tests, but they do it in triplicate and run it two separate times in the production process!

I've included a list of the tests below, and a brief definition, you are welcome to look up each one of them and see what they do in further detail.

Densitometry – Measures the density of a liquid

Viscometry – Measures the viscosity of a liquid

Refractometry – Measures the refractive index of a liquid or solid sample

Olfactometry – Detects and measures odor dilution

Polarimetry – Measures the angle of rotation caused by passing polarized light through an optically active substance

Inductively Coupled Plasma Mass Spectrometry (ICP-MS) – Measures elements on the basis of their mass to charge ratio

Inductively Coupled Plasma-Atomic Optical Emission Spectrometry (ICP-OES) – An analytical technique used for the detection of chemical elements

Gas Chromatography (GC) – Separates a mixture of molecules into individual chemicals and then determines the amount of each chemical

High Performance Liquid Chromatography (HPLC) – Used to separate, identify, and quantify each component in a mixture

Fourier Transform Infrared Spectroscopy – Used to obtain an infrared spectrum of absorption or emission of a solid, liquid or gas

Automated Micro-Enumeration – Method used to estimate microbial populations

Accelerated Stability Testing – Measures degradation of a product stored at elevated stress conditions (such as temperature, humidity, and pH)

Disintegration – Measures, under standard conditions, the ability of a sample to break into smaller particles

pH – Measure of the acidity or alkalinity of a solution

Microscopy – Determines the microstructure or nanostructure of materials, chemicals or products

Combustibility – Determines the degree of flammability

Flash Point – Checks for contamination or adulteration of product

Water Activity – Used to predict the stability and safety of food with respect to microbial growth, rates of deteriorative reactions and chemical/physical properties

Gas Chromatography Mass Spectrometry (GCMS) – Analytical method that combines the features of gas-chromatography and mass spectrometry to identify different substances within a test sample by separating chemical mixtures and identifies the components at a molecular level

Chiral Chromatography – Used to separate and identify complex mixtures and analyzes the 3-dimensional structure of molecules

Isotope Ratio Mass Spectrometry (IRMS) – Measures the relative abundance of isotopes in a given sample.

Knowing that Young Living cares about the quality and purity of the product, so much that they run these 21 tests, gives me even greater assurance on the Seed to Seal® guarantee.

Research & Development

Since quality and purity have always been uncompromising standards and values for D. Gary Young, and Young Living throughout the years, the science, equipment, scientists and laboratories to test and verify the purity have also been greatly valued and supported.

Gary loved to teach people, and personally trained over 50 scientists, passing on not only how to perform the rigorous duties of quality testing, research, and development, but also his vision, desire to care for others and his solid commitment to unwavering quality. These scientists in turn have absorbed his approach, wisdom, and intentions towards developing new Young Living products.

D. Gary Young was the father of the modern-day essential oils movement, and left a legacy and vision in the hearts of those he trained. They are forever and fully infused into the product research and development efforts. As a continual reminder of Gary's vision, expertise, and uncompromising standards and values of quality and purity, Young Living's Research and Development team was renamed the D. Gary Young Research Institute in June 2018, and they uphold his vision.

As always, Young Living only allows uncompromisingly pure, therapeutic grade essential oils into product formulas and oil-infused products, and doesn't allow products to include parabens, artificial colors or dyes, nitrates, GMOs, or phthalates, or undergo animal testing.

Since only the purest ingredients go into Young Living's products, you can be sure that the products you are using are safe for your family, no matter where you are using them in your home.

The Standards, and especially the Science pillar, from the Seed to Seal® quality commitment, are infused into every molecule of the D. Gary Young Research Institute. Utilizing innovative product development, quality standards, rigorous research, and cutting-edge methods, the scientific staff, led by Chief Science Officer Dr. Michael Buch, ensure the quality, purity, and efficacy of all Young Living's products, while researching and developing unique new products that lead the industry.

OTC Products

Young Living's over-the-counter (OTC) products are created in state-of-the-art labs with some of the most advanced scientific equipment available, where the D. Gary Young Research Institute develops new testing methods that support product claims and uses while ensuring quality, purity and efficacy.

These products have undergone rigorous testing, and have been approved for OTC usage. Since they are approved for OTC drug use, they are allowed to make claims.

Below are some of the products included in their new OTC product line and the claims they can legally make!

- **Young Living's Cool Azul™ Pain Relief Cream** – provides cooling relief from minor muscle and joint aches, arthritis, strains, bruises, and sprains. With two powerful, synergistic active ingredients, this cream provides pain-relieving benefits in two ways: methyl salicylate found in Wintergreen helps alleviate pain deep in the muscles and joints, and natural menthol found in Peppermint provides a cooling effect.

- **Seedlings™ Diaper Rash Cream** – Made with 100 percent naturally derived ingredients, including 100 percent pure essential oils. This thick, Lavender-scented cream reduces the duration and severity of diaper rash when applied at the first sign of redness.

It soothes on contact, protects your baby's delicate skin, and acts as a physical barrier to wetness.

- **LavaDerm™ After-Sun Spray** – This naturally derived after-sun spray offers temporary relief from the pain and itching of minor burns, minor cuts, sunburns, scrapes, insect bites, and minor skin irritations, so your family can keep playing all day.

- **Insect Repellent** – Tested to repel mosquitoes, ticks, and fleas using only 100 percent naturally derived, plant-based ingredients.

- **Maximum-Strength Acne Treatment** – Naturally derived, maximum-strength salicylic acid from Wintergreen helps clear acne blemishes, pimples, and blackheads; but its plant-based powers don't stop there! Tca Tree essential oil helps cleanse your skin, while Manuka oil reduces the appearance of blemishes.

- **Mineral Sunscreen Lotion SPF 10** – Provides protection against UVA and UVB rays without harsh chemical ingredients. Instead, the non-greasy sunscreen offers broad-spectrum SPF 10 protection using naturally derived plant- and mineral-based ingredients, including non- nano zinc oxide—a physical UV blocker.

- **Mineral Sunscreen Lotion SPF 50** – This natural sunscreen is chemical-free, making it a healthy alternative for adults and kids! Instead of melting in the sun, melt this lightweight, fast-absorbing sunscreen into your skin for added protection from UVA and UVB rays.

- **Thieves® Essential Oil Infused Cough Drops** – The power of Thieves® and menthol in a cough drop! The triple-action formula of Thieves® Cough Drops offers comfort by relieving coughs, soothing sore throats, and cooling nasal passages.

It is very refreshing that, in a world of compliance, the OTC products give us an ability to speak about Young Living with approved and verified product claims.

Proof In Action – Check The Facts

After reading about Testing & Standards, you might want a cheat sheet to remember all of the specifics and nuances.

No Compromising
- Young Living would rather go without an essential oil than compromise on quality.
- Young Living is a company that will not compromise on quality no matter how much profit is involved.

Testing Before Harvesting & Distillation
- BRIX testing done in the weeks and days leading up to harvest to figure out when the plant is ready to be harvested.
- Small, test distills are also done to determine therapeutic properties of new plants.

Types & Number Of Tests
- Young Living also performs 21 different tests on their essential oils to ensure that its members receive the highest quality essential oils in the world!
- Not only do they perform 21 separate tests, but they do it in triplicate and run it two separate times in the production process.

Research & Development
- Since quality and purity have always been uncompromising standards and values for D. Gary Young, and his legacy lives on through the people he trained.

- The three pillars of the Seed to Seal® process, Sourcing, Science, and Standards.

OTC Products

- State of the art products with allowed claims made possible through rigorous testing and more than 50 well trained scientists.

In the next chapter, we will be learning about sustainability and education, and how Young Living continues to grow, predict the future needs and teach members useful skills and tips.

CHAPTER 6

Sustainability & Education

"Your money is power, so be aware of the products you're buying and the companies you're supporting to make sure you're helping the companies that are leading the way in sustainability."
~Gretchen Bleiler

Sustainability

The core of Young Living has always been about sustainability. By sustainably producing the highest quality essential oils on the planet through the three pillars of Sourcing, Science and Standards, Young Living is able to provide a sustained impact on the daily lives of individuals for the better with a toxin-free lifestyle, and empower those in need through the Young Living Foundation.

In my opinion, one of the first lessons that Gary received on this was when he was told by a mentor, "If you don't grow it, the time will come when you won't be able to distill it!"

He realized having his own farms was very important, not only to be able to guarantee the quality and purity of his essential oils, but to ensure that he had a sustainable resource that would grow as his company's needs increased.

To honor Gary and propel his vision forward for the next 5 years, Young Living created 5 pledges to sustain Gary's desire to constantly change lives for the better and provide a toxin-free lifestyle to everyone on the planet.

Starting in 2019, and over the next 5 years, Young Living has dedicated itself to fulfill this 5 x 5 pledge.

- 5 times the lives empowered by the D. Gary Young, Young Living Foundation
- 5 or more new markets opened each year
- 5 million additional households reached
- 5 years to zero waste
- 5 or more new corporate farms or partner farms developed each year

While Young Living already has a huge impact on the lives of individuals with the D. Gary Young, Young Living Foundation, the growth of the company into more markets will only enable them to empower, save and support more individuals in the future.

Furthermore, while Young Living is working on creating more corporate owned and partner farms, the quality, selection and purity of essential oils provided will only increase as well, because Young Living never settles for lower quality essential oils!

What an incredible legacy that Young Living will leave to empower the lives of millions of people, continue to reduce their negative impact on the environment, and create more resources for the highest quality essential oils on the planet.

International Grand Convention

The International Grand Convention is the single largest event for Young Living every year, and brings people from every corner of the world. In 2018, there were over 30,000 people in attendance and, amazingly, there are more every year. I can't think of a time when I've seen that many people in one location over a four-day event, and on day four people are still smiling, joyful, and happy like one big family.

The main focus of the International Grand Convention is of course the general session, where there is teaching, training, and instruction of new products from corporate staff, executive officers, and science officers. The main highlights of the general session are the new product reveals and the amazing motivational speakers leading us in self-improvement and self-growth.

At past general sessions, I've learned things like how I'm limiting myself, how my attitude, vision, and gratitude affect my reaching of goals, and how the best methods for being productive every day include starting my day with purpose and living each day with intention.

While the keynote speakers are amazing, and world-changing, and learning about new products is awesome, some of my favorite parts of the convention are meeting other people, talking to team members and being able to connect with like-minded people on a personal level. Not only that, but being able to meet with corporate staff, and the executive team, really keeps the atmosphere feeling like a giant caring family where everyone is there to help.

There are plenty of opportunities to be able to have impromptu meetings with friends and other individuals you meet in the hallways, and you can always see what topics of interest are available at the breakout sessions. The NingXia Red® Bar in the product expo, for custom NingXia Red® mixes, is also an excellent place to talk to others and enjoy some amazing refreshment as well!

Besides the general session, another favorite for everyone is the Farm Day Experience. At the farm you get to live the Seed to Seal® quality commitment in person, and work in the fields to plant seedlings, tour the distillery, harvest some lavender, and visit with the world famous Percheron draft horses. The farm is truly a wonderful experience and Young Living goes all out. There is also a barbecue, jousting tournament, and something for everyone.

Other events that happen at the International Grand Convention that help to foster team unity are: the opening and closing parties, the warehouse tour, the call-center tour, the global headquarters tour, scavenger hunts and opportunities to learn from veteran oilers.

Young Living's International Grand Convention is something that everyone should go to!

Podcasts & Videos

Young Living's training and education team is a wonderful resource for learning how to use essential oil products, and especially any new products that are created. The Young Living Education and Training team does an excellent job of recording videos and podcasts filled with essential oil tips, DIYs, recipes, science, and other ways of infusing your life with Young Living products. Their invaluable posts are provided daily, and are full of tips, tricks, education on products, as well as interviews with veteran oilers and other experts.

The veteran oilers provide information on how best to support a particular body system, share their favorite products and uses, and even provide sharing tips.

When there is a guest appearance by Chief Science Officer Dr. Michael Buch, I especially love sitting and listening to the wisdom he provides on the creation, testing and use of essential oils and essential oil products.

Last but not least, after the convention every summer, where there are usually many new Young Living products released, the Young Living Education and Training group produces a video on each of the products. Users can learn how best to use the new products, and also learn any tips and tricks that the Education and Training team has already learned by using the products.

Beauty School

Multiple times a year, Young Living hosts a Beauty School where people, mostly women, from all over the world come to not only get first-hand knowledge of how best to utilize the Young Living products in their beauty routines, but to learn the best products, procedures and method of cleansing their faces, and even how to apply makeup to highlight their best features.

These classes and instructional period are filled with wisdom from women who have used these products for years, and know the best way to cleanse and support their skin.

My wife, Carrie, has been truly thankful for the changes that it has made in her beauty routine, and feels more confident in her selection and use of the products, and really loves the instruction and training on Savvy Mineral Makeup.

As wonderful as all that is, the real gem of beauty school to me seems to be the other content given from the presenters. The presenters uplift and encourage the women and help them to find and accentuate their best qualities and inner strengths, and feel more beautiful.

My wife, who is already an exceptional woman and full of beauty, has been to several Beauty School events, but always seems to come back with a greater understanding of her inner beauty, and a greater self-knowledge and purpose. What seems to flood away is the false image of beauty that is portrayed in magazines, on billboards and TV, and when she returns home, she is better able to see her God-given beauty and purpose.

I watched this phenomenon happen for at least 2 years before my eldest daughter went with my wife, and my daughter also came home bubbling with excitement, an inner purpose, and a knowledge of her own beauty! What she had been told all along now seems to radiate from her eyes.

I know that beauty school is not a women's only event, but I have never had a chance to talk to any of the guys that have gone, so I don't know what their take away is.

Live Your Passion Rallies

The Live Your Passion Rally is a way to experience everything about Young Living in one location, through content-rich presentations, product sampling and information, personal conversation, exciting announcements, training and business-building tools.

This event is a quarterly event that is hosted by other Young Living members in your area, and supported by Young

Living, who provides the majority of the content presented, but individual hosts are encouraged to add their own local flair.

The most recent rally had over 2,800 hosts in 40 countries that brought together over 150,000 people around the globe. The members host the meetings because they simply love talking about their oils, and inspiring more people to live a life of wellness, purpose and abundance.

So find out when the next Live Your Passion Rally is near you and join in on the fun!

Proof In Action – Check The Facts

This chapter is really about how Young Living cares for you, while also caring for the environment, and the cost is worth it for Sustainability & Education.

Sustainability

- Having your own farms is very important, because if you grow it you can distill it.
- Guarantee quality and purity of essential oils, throughout the whole process.
- Ensure a stainable resource that will grow as the company's needs increase.
- 5 pledges to sustain Gary's desire to constantly change lives for the better and provide a toxin-free lifestyle to everyone on the planet.

International Grand Convention

- Meet the real people involved in the company's process, planning and direction.
- Experience Seed to Seal® first hand and participate in the process.
- Receive amazing teaching, training and mentoring on products and for self-growth.

Podcasts & Videos

- Videos and podcasts filled with essential oil tips, DIYs, recipes, science, and other ways of infusing your life with Young Living products.

- Daily invaluable posts are full of tips, tricks, and education on products.
- Interviews with veteran oilers, teach how best to support a particular body system, share their favorite products and uses, and even provide sharing tips.

Beauty School

- Learn how best to utilize Young Living products in beauty routines.
- Understand best products, procedures and method of cleansing face.
- Receive education on how to apply makeup to highlight your best features.
- Find greater understanding of inner beauty, greater self- knowledge, and purpose.

Live Your Passion Rallies

- Experience everything about Young Living in one location, through content-rich presentations, product sampling and information.
- Engage in personal conversation, hear exciting announcements, and learn training and sharing tools.

Now that we have learned about Young Living's passion on sustainable growth, farms, and continued education, I hope you have a better understanding of how much care Young Living puts into you! In the next chapter, we will see what is near and dear to the heart of Young Living as we follow the money again!

CHAPTER 7

Follow The Money Again

"The highest use of capital is not to make more money, but to make money do more for the betterment of life."
~Henry Ford

The Young Living Academy

While there are different ways of following the money with Young Living, I believe the most world-changing and impactful way is through the D. Gary Young, Young Living Foundation. The Young Living Foundation was started by D. Gary Young because he saw a need, and decided to do something to fulfill that need.

While he was building the farm in Guayaquil, Ecuador, Gary passed a cracked and broken down building every day on his way to the farm, and eventually started to see a lot of different children around this building. He stopped and investigated, and found out that the building was a one-room schoolhouse, with 42 students, ranging from 1st-6th grade, all in the same room, being taught by one volunteer teacher, with little to no materials. His heart broke.

He knew he had to do something, so he worked with local leaders, and after buying a section of land and starting construction on the new schoolhouse, he had the school transfer there and the Young Living Academy started with 83 students. Gary started the Young Living Foundation to build the school, hire teachers, provide textbooks, meals and even scholarships for students to be able to attend and eventually graduate high school. In a country where most students drop out by the eighth grade, this school allowed them to graduate high school and attend college to become doctors, lawyers and engineers!

Instead of an easily flooded, broken down one-room schoolhouse with one volunteer teacher and outdoor bathroom sheds the Young Living Academy occupied a building on high ground, with teachers for every grade, was two stories tall, had indoor plumbing, electricity and teaching supplies.

When I first visited the school in 2014, it was a two-story building with one wing and a long low building for the younger grades. When I went back in 2016, it still had the long one-story building, but the two-story building now had two wings, including a computer lab and music room, a sports field, and a covered gymnasium. Additionally, that year was the year of the first high-school graduating class with 12 students, and an unheard of 100% graduation rate! Now the Young Living Academy has over 350 students ranging from Pre-K through 12th grade and has had 4 years of graduating classes, the latest with 21 students!

The mission and vision of the D. Gary Young, Young Living Foundation is to empower individuals to achieve their potential, and provide children with the opportunities necessary to become self- reliant individuals who can take charge control over their own health, provide for their families and positively change their communities.

The Foundation surely has met its goals with the Young Living Academy. Let's take a moment to look at all the rest of the projects it serves.

Administrative Costs & Rounding

Young Living Essential Oils completely covers all administrative costs; 100% of the donations given to the Young Living Foundation go directly to the individuals in need, and to the carefully selected partnerships and projects.

Young Living members also have the opportunity to choose to round up every one of their orders to the nearest dollar. Last year, $1.1 million was raised, and all the money went to the Young Living Foundation, to be sent to projects like the Young Living Academy and lifesaving partnerships.

Rebuilding Nepal

In April 2015 a massive 7.8 magnitude earthquake occurred in Nepal, killing 9,000 people, injuring 22,000 and leaving nearly 3.5 million people homeless. Nine months later, Gary visited Nepal and was overwhelmed with the devastation that still existed. He knew that the mountain villages would be harder hit, and aide would be less able to travel in over the tenuous mountain roads.

He traveled to Yarsa, Nepal, the epicenter of the quake, and found a mountain village of 100 homes and a school totally destroyed, with sub-zero temperatures and heavy rains making their makeshift shelters painfully inadequate.

Gary had this to say about the situation when he arrived, "We were the first to bring help with a semi load of blankets, coats, sweaters, hats, and pajamas. Handing out the supplies to every member of the village was a very emotional and gut-wrenching experience. The week before I arrived, 24 people had died from exposure, and two children died while I was there handing out the blankets."

Gary returned with the Young Living Foundation, purchased a complete automated block factory from South Africa and shipped it to Yarsa. This provided jobs for more than 50 local people and utilized one of the resources that Yarsa that had in abundance, mud!

This machine makes bricks from dirt mixed with a small amount of cement. It is very easy to operate, seismic safe, and efficient; and the bricks are very inexpensive because of their composite ingredients.

The Young Living Foundation provided the funds to purchase the brick-making factory, and led service trips to Nepal to work building houses. Because of their donation and efforts, as of July 2018, all 100 homes had been rebuilt in Yarsa!

Hope For Justice

The Young Living Foundation has partnered with Hope for Justice to end one of the biggest problems in our world today, human trafficking. More than half of the 20 million slaves are women and girls.

Hope for Justice uses the funds provided to follow a four-tiered strategy to bring freedom to the lost.

> **1.** **Train**: They train the police, doctors, outreach programs and other professionals on the front lines to identify victims.

2. **Rescue**: After identifying victims of human trafficking, they remove them from the situations of exploitation by building bridges of trust.

3. **Advocate**: They advocate for the victims' access to housing and health services while securing criminal and civil justice for the victims and cancelling trafficker created debts.

4. **Restore**: Their restorative care home and programs help victims overcome trauma and rebuild their lives.

More than 90 percent of victims who are rescued by Hope for Justice and its programs never return to trafficking, giving Hope for Justice the highest success rate of nonprofits battling modern-day slavery.

Sole Hope

The Young Living Foundation has partnered with Sole Hope to provide resources and services to allow men, women and children who live in sub-Saharan climates to become and remain jigger free. Jiggers are sand fleas, parasitic insects that lie relatively undetected on the dirt floors of homes and schools in Uganda and burrow into the hands and feet of barefoot adults and children.

Young Living, with the help of the Young Living Foundation, held shoe cutting parties throughout the United States to prepare all the donated raw materials for shipment to Uganda. The parties overwhelmingly provided all the materials Sole Hope would need for the next year and more.

These shoes are made from old blue jeans and plastic milk jugs, and the soles are made from old tires, ensuring that the shoes won't wear out before the child outgrows them.

Additionally, the D. Gary Young, Young Living Foundation is helping provide funds for Sole Hope to purchase land and build a new outreach house in Jinja, Uganda. The outreach house is a place where jigger infected individuals can stay, receive treatment, healing and education on jiggers, and other areas of life including laundry, cooking and crafts.

Healing Faith Uganda

The D. Gary Young, Young Living Foundation partnered with Healing Faith Uganda in 2015 to fight against malaria in Eastern Uganda. In Africa, one person dies every minute from malaria, and the majority of those deaths are children under five.

The malaria education, prevention and treatment to families and children by Healing Faith Uganda is invaluable since they focus on the smaller, more remote villages with little outside access to aid.

The Young Living Foundation was able to purchase over 4,000 mosquito nets with funds raised at the Young Living 2015 international Grand Convention, and several members went on a humanitarian trip with Healing Faith Uganda to deliver the donation. They were able to cover every bed in the entire village of Wasaki with all the nets purchased!

The incredible support by the donors to the Young Living Foundation has increased the amount of $5 mosquito nets from 400 nets per month to more than 4,000. This means that the Young Living Foundation is responsible for over a 1,000 percent impact increase in the work of Healing Faith Uganda.

Disaster Relief

The D. Gary Young, Young Living Foundation is always ready to lend a hand to those in need, even those who are affected by natural disasters.

In October 2018, Michael, the first Category 4 hurricane to hit the Florida Panhandle, destroyed many homes and businesses. Young Living Foundation Ambassadors coordinated efforts, driving to Panama City Beach, Florida and other affected communities, and distributed supplies. Additionally, the Young Living Foundation donated $5,000 to support efforts in cleaning muck out of homes, sealing roofs with tarps, and bringing together skilled electricians to those still without power.

In November, 2018, the Camp Fire became the deadliest and most destructive wildfire in California's history. In the aftermath of the fires, the Young Living Foundation donated over $23,000 worth of fire kits that contained essential oils and other products, to affected members and community organizations in the Paradise area.

In September 2017, an earthquake reduced countless homes to rubble in Puebla, Mexico, and injured over 6,000 people. Almost a year later, the Young Living Foundation was able to team up with Young Living Mexico members and staff, and the non-profit organization, Techo, to identify those still in need, and rebuild homes.

This is just a few of the ways that the D. Gary Young, Young Living Foundation supports those in need and is ready to lend a hand. Young Living Essential Oils makes that possible by paying 100% of the Foundation's administrative costs, sending generous donations to the Foundation, and providing ways for its members to donate as well.

Proof In Action – Check The Facts

After learning about the Heart of Young Living, here are some bullet points on each of the Young Living Foundation areas.

The Young Living Academy

- Young Living Foundation was started by D. Gary Young because he saw children in need, and decided to do something about it to fulfill that need.
- Young Living completely covers the Foundation's administrative costs.
- 100% of Young Living Foundation donations go directly to individuals in need.
- Last year, Young Living members raised $1.1 million just by rounding up orders.
- Young Living Academy has 350 students, Pre-K - 12th grade, and a 100% graduation rate.

Rebuilding Nepal

- Yarsa, Nepal, a mountain village of 100 homes and the epicenter of the quake, was still totally destroyed 9 months later.
- Young Living Foundation paid for and shipped a complete automated block factory.
- As of July 2018, service trips to Nepal rebuilt all 100 homes in Yarsa.

Hope For Justice

- Hope for Justice partnered to end human trafficking of more than 20 million slaves.
- Funds provided to follow a four-tiered strategy to bring freedom: Train, Rescue, Advocate, and Restore.
- More than 90 percent of victims rescued by Hope for Justice and its programs never return to trafficking.

Sole Hope

- Provides resources and services to allow men, women and children who live in sub-Saharan climates to become and remain jigger free.
- Donated high quality shoes that won't wear out before the child outgrows them.

Healing Faith Uganda

- Increased amount of $5 mosquito nets from 400 nets per month to more than 4,000.
- Responsible for over 1,000% impact increase in the work of Healing Faith Uganda.

Disaster Relief

- Always ready to lend a hand to those affected by natural disasters worldwide.
- Provided supplies and workers to help with the cleanup for hurricanes, fires, and earthquakes.

To figure out what a business cares about, look into how they spend their time and money. In the next chapter, I will talk more about how Young Living spends its money on Compliance & Rewards, as well as its integrity and benefits.

CHAPTER 8

Compliance & Rewards

"With integrity, you have nothing to fear, since you have nothing to hide. With integrity, you will do the right thing, so you will have no guilt."
~Zig Ziglar

Compliance, The FDA, & Vague Descriptions

Why don't Young Living essential oils product brochures talk plainly about what their products do? Why are their words intentionally vague? Why do they have to include the disclaimer, "This statement has not been evaluated by the Food and Drug Administration. This product is not intended to diagnose, treat, cure, or prevent any disease."?

The answer is, essential oil companies are not allowed to, no matter how effective their products really are, make a claim that would be considered a drug claim.

The Food and Drug Administration (FDA) declares, "Only a drug can cure, prevent, or treat a disease." The absurdity of this is evident if you take a look at aspirin. Even though it was originally created using the chemical structure of the willow tree, aspirin can make many drug claims about its effects and properties, but the same claims can not be made about a product made from the willow tree, or the FDA would have to regulate all willow trees.

Because "only a drug can cure, prevent, or treat a disease," products that claim to have an effect on any disease are considered drugs by the FDA, and are strictly regulated.

Essential oils therefore fit into the dietary supplements category. What this means is, the FDA doesn't allow Young Living or any independent distributors to make disease claims; in other words, to claim that an essential oil will cure, treat or prevent any disease. What is left for Young Living and all essential oil companies is to make one of 4 types of claims, **Health Claims, Nutritional Claims, Claims of Well-Being,** and **Structure or Function Claims**.

Health Claims require the approval of the FDA and include something like "Calcium may reduce the risk of osteoporosis."

However, Nutritional Claims, Claims of Well-Being and Structure Function Claims do NOT require the approval of the FDA, but do require the use of the obligatory disclaimer.

"This statement has not been evaluated by the Food and Drug Administration. This product is not intended to diagnose, treat, cure, or prevent any disease."

This statement does not mean the products are somehow less effective, or that the company is lying to hide something; instead the use of this statement means that the company using it is actually following the law. This statement is required after having made a Nutritional Claim, Claim of Well- Being or Structure Function Claim.

Nutritional Claims are statements like "XYZ product is a good source of calcium, which means XYZ has at least 15% of the recommended daily intake of calcium."

Claims of Well-Being are statements like "This product improves your mood."

Structure Function Claims are statements that fall under one of a few select categories. The following examples were taken from the website www.cancer.org.

- The product's mechanism of action ("works as an antioxidant")
- The product's effects on cellular structure ("helps membrane stability")
- The product's effects on the body's physiology ("promotes normal urinary flow")
- The product's effects on chemical or lab test results ("supports normal blood glucose")
- Claims of maintenance ("helps maintain a healthy circulatory system")
- Other non-disease claims ("helps you relax")
- Claims for common conditions and symptoms related to life stages ("reduces irritability, bloating, and cramping associated with premenstrual syndrome")

Young Living Essential Oils is a company dedicated to following the law, has policies and procedures in place to meet these standards, and has followed the rules on their websites, printed materials and distributor training materials.

The Lacey Act of 1900

Apart from the FDA, there are many other laws that an essential oil company has to follow, one of which is the Lacey

Act. The Lacey Act was originally created in 1900 to monitor the unlawful sale or possession of plants, fish and wildlife, but was expanded in 2008 to include a wider variety of prohibited plants and plant products.

Young Living realized in 2014 that they may have unintentionally violated this law, so they removed the products from sale in their inventory, and began an internal investigation. In 2015, the internal investigation told them that they had violated the Lacey Act in regards to Rosewood and Spikenard. Knowing that they would face a fine, Young Living stood with integrity and approached the Department of Justice and voluntarily disclosed their discovered sourcing issue, which began an investigation.

Young Living worked with the government and developed a sourcing plan to that meet the stringent requirements of the Lacey Act and is currently the only essential oil company with a Lacey Act Compliance Plan. Additionally, when Young Living is looking to find new partner farms, they bring an independent Environmental Watch Group, SPF Global, with them to make sure they stay in compliance.

The investigation resulting from self-reporting led to a court date, at which Young Living pled guilty and paid a fine of $500,000, in addition to $135,000 in restitution and a $125,000 community service payment for protected plants conservation.

Why does this show that Young Living is the best essential oil company? Because when they unknowingly violated the law, they reported themselves. That shows a company with integrity, doing the right thing, even though they knew that they would be prosecuted and fined.

They are the only essential oil company with a Lacey Act Compliance plan in place, and have stopped selling Rosewood and Spikenard, while other companies are still selling them. With no sustainable source for either product, how many essential oil companies are breaking the Lacey Act Compliance and not reporting?

Young Living acted with integrity, by doing what was right, despite the cost, even when no one was looking, and any company willing to do that makes them the best company.

Beyond the FDA and Lacey Act compliance, Young Living takes it one step further and makes sure their products are Conflict Free. Conflict Free is a self-imposed requirement that Young Living follows to make sure that their raw materials are not sourced from areas of violence, war, or human rights violations. Purchasing products from Young Living means you can rest your conscience and know that the products were ethically sourced and are the highest quality products on the planet.

Knowing and following the FDA rules on compliance regarding disease claims, the rules and tenants of the Lacey Act, and Conflict Free sourcing are three more factors that set Young Living apart from every essential oil.

Ask Yourself...
Does your company have any policies and procedures in place to comply with the FDA regulations on making disease claims? Do they import and sell any essential oils from rare and endangered species? Rosewood? Spikenard? Do they have any policies and procedures in place to make sure that your sourcing is from verifiable accepted sources and doesn't break any laws or treaties? Are their products Conflict Free?

Why Network Marketing Makes Sense

As I mentioned in an earlier chapter, there are people who are against network marketing companies just because it is a network marketing company. I explained that many of the complaints are based on the belief that because it is a network marketing company, they are paying higher prices in order for the company to be able to pay their distributors. That makes sense for some network marketing companies, but for Young Living the increased prices really are due to the greatly increased quality, testing and standards!

As we talked about earlier, a true measure of the quality and standards of an essential oil company can be found simply by looking at the price and distillation procedures of Rose Essential Oil. For Young Living, the distillation of Rose Essential Oil takes 2,000 lbs of rose petals to make one gallon, or 200 lbs of rose petals for one 5 ml bottle of Rose Essential Oil.

Earlier I also talked about the research and development of Idaho Balsam Fir Essential Oil, and how it took Young Living 7 years to figure out how to get the greatest amount of therapeutic properties from Idaho Balsam Fir.

Finally, we talked about the dedication to sourcing, science, and standards that encompasses the three pillars of Young Living's Seed to Seal® Quality, the commitment to following federal and international laws and treaties, and all of the testing performed to meet all of those requirements, and we came to the conclusion that quality is worth paying for!

But I'll humor you for a moment, and talk about the costs associated with paying distributors for network marketing.

In the first five years, most startup companies spend between 10% and 20% on marketing and branding, just to get the word out about themselves, but 50% of startup companies fail in the first five years. What good does all that spending do for you if people are still not buying your products?

It seems to me that new companies, especially ones with awesome quality, would want to spend their marketing money in the most effective way. Research shows that word-of-mouth marketing is the most effective form of advertising and marketing.

If word-of-mouth advertising accounts for generating five times the sales of paid media impressions or advertising, and people are 90% more likely to buy a product if recommended by a friend, then wouldn't it make sense to focus on word-of-mouth advertising? Network marketing is essentially word-of-mouth advertising.

When was the last time you tried a new ice cream flavor at a local ice cream shop and told all your friends that they had to go try it? Did the store pay you for advertising for them? My guess is no, but Young Living does! Young Living sends a thank you check to people who share with their friends about what they love!

When Young Living was a new company, and as a direct result of Gary's experience, it started out with an exceptional product and decided to use this factor to its advantage by utilizing the single most effective form of marketing and advertising by paying people for the referrals with network marketing. So that is what Young Living still does today. They do not sell in grocery stores, but rather sell exclusively by word-of-mouth advertising. With over $1.9 billion in sales annually, Young Living must be doing something right!

Ask Yourself...

Have you ever talked about something you loved with a friend or family member? Would you like to get a thank you check for sharing what you love?

The Accidental Paycheck

I know what you're thinking, how can someone receive an accidental paycheck? I'll tell you how!

When we were supporting our daughter Jubilee's health, and my wife, Carrie, was oiling Jubilee's feet, Carrie decided to oil her mom's feet as well. My mother-in-law was visiting to help us through this time and happened to be sitting right next to Jubliee, and while she looked up curiously at Carrie when she got oils put on her feet, she laughed and thought nothing of it.

About 15 minutes later, my mother-in-law jumped off couch and exclaimed, "I don't know what those things are, but I want some! I feel amazing!" We muddled through how to get her a starter kit and a few more oils and products she wanted to try, and thought no more of the event.

About three weeks later, we got a check from Young Living for $76.93, and couldn't figure out what it was! After calling our friend, we found out that Young Living had sent us a thank you check for showing my mother-in-law how to get what she wanted. Wow, an accidental paycheck!

Would you like to get an accidental paycheck for sharing what you love?

Another way to follow the money in Young Living is of course the Young Living Compensation Plan, where they pay their distributors. So how does it work?

The Compensation Plan has many parts, and Young Living has many videos in the Virtual Office that explain the many parts in detail, so I will simply focus on the first part that applies to the accidental paycheck, the bonuses. If you would like more on the compensation plan, there will be a link provided in the Proof In Action section at the end of this chapter and in the bonus material available on the book website, TheBestEO.com.

For more detailed books on the Young Living Compensation Plan look for the following titles:
- *Grow : Seeds of Wisdom For Budding Leaders*, Amanda Uribe.
- *Gameplan : The Complete Strategy Guide to go from Starter Kit to Silver*, Sarah Harnisch.
- *Driven For Success : Road Map to the Comp Plan*, Jake Dempsey.

Below is a sample of how sharing with your friends what you love can get you an accidental paycheck and even pay for your kit.

The bonuses include the Premium Starter Kit (PSK) bonus for $25 and the Fast Start bonus for 25% of a new signup's Personal Volume (PV) (or as I look at it, Product Value) for the first 3 months.

All of the PSKs are worth 100PV, whether it be the PSK (Essential Oils), the PSK with Thieves®, the PSK with NingXia or the PSK with Savvy Minerals.

So let's say you sign up with the PSK in January, start to use your essential oils and starter kit samples, love them and share about these cool new products with three friends, Zeke, Abby and Beth. You share about how you are impressed with the Seed to Seal® quality, the essential oils you love to

use after a workout, how you like the smell of the Thieves®
Cleaner, and how a NingXia Red® helped you recover from
your workout with energy.

Now Zeke hears about how much you loved the Thieves®
Cleaner sample in your starter kit and decides to order the
PSK with Thieves® because he loves the sound of replacing
all the toxic cleaners in his house. He orders a total of 100PV.

Abby hears about how much you loved your products,
likes the Seed to Seal® promise and decides to buy the PSK
with Savvy Minerals (100PV), because she loves the idea of
using a makeup without talc, bismuth, parabens, phthalates,
petrochemicals, or synthetic fragrances. She also decides to
get on Essential Rewards, tosses in a 15ml of Copaiba (44.25
PV) and PanAway® (81.75 PV) after hearing how much you
loved them on your joints after a workout, and says she is
going to use ER to try new products every month. She orders
a total of 226 PV.

Beth sees how much energy you had after trying the
NingXia Red® from your starter kit and wants some of that
energy for herself! She decides to go with the PSK with
Ningxia and decides to get on essential rewards to keep
Ningxia available in her home. She orders a total of 100PV.

Your estimated Accidental Paycheck would be:

PSK bonus for Zeke	$25.00
Fast start bonus for Zeke	$25.00
PSK Bonus for Abby	$25.00
Fast start bonus for Abby	$56.50
PSK Bonus for Beth	$25.00
Fast start bonus for Beth	$25.00
Total Bonuses for January	**$181.50**

All you did was talk about the things you love and were impressed with, and your friends wanted to try it too. Just like you would do with that new ice cream flavor, but in this case, you got paid for sharing what you love.

Does that mean that you have to make it a business? Nope, there is no requirement to build a business. You can just keep using the products and support your family's health, but don't be surprised if you find yourself sharing more about what you love.

Getting Paid To Shop In My Own Store

One of my most favorite things about Young Living is getting paid to shop in my own store. Young Living has a program called the Essential Rewards (ER) program, and it is an optional program for people who want to order monthly with at least a 50 PV order. For about 95% of the products in the YL catalog, $1 spent equals 1 PV.

The remaining 5% are the exceptions, which include the membership enrollment kits, which are already such a fantasticdeal, the three most expensive oils that Young Living makes, any brand new products, and any non-essential oil products such as catalogs, info booklets, bottle labels, and empty gel capsules.

So how do I get paid for shopping in my own store? Essential Rewards is Young Living's Loyalty Rewards program through which they pay percentage of your order back to you in points.

Months 1-3	10% back in points
Months 4-24	20% back in points
Months 25+	25% back in points

What does this mean? Well, for simplicity's sake I'm going to use a 100 PV order. My first month, I decide to sign up with a membership kit and ER. I choose the option to have the membership kit qualify for my ER order for my first month, and since it is worth 100 PV, I get back 10 points. My second month, I decide to spend a 100 PV order, I get back 10 points. My third month I decide to spend a 100 PV order and I also get back 10 points. After three months of being on ER, I'm now allowed to cash in my points and I already have a total of 30 points. I can now place an order that would cost me $30 for 30 PV worth of product and cash in my points and only pay shipping.

I just got paid $30 worth of product, just for shopping in my own store!

Additionally, for making a 100 PV ER order, I receive a bonus essential oil every month. Young Living usually has freebies at different price points, and since I transferred my buying from toxin laden products in the grocery store to Young Living's awesome toxin-free products, I can spend the money I would have spent elsewhere and save even more money while supporting my family's health.

Traditionally, there is an ER exclusive bonus oil for spending 100 PV and also at 250PV, but I can also receive other free oils and products at 190PV, 250PV, 300PV and sometimes even 400PV or 500PV. Even better, all the non-ER bonus products received for placing an order of 190 PV, 250 PV and 300PV (or higher), I can receive a second time with 1 non-ER order per month as well. That means, on average, I earn between $80-$120 of free products per order or up to $160-$240 per month.

Lastly, Young Living gives me a free gift for consecutive orders at 3, 6, 9 & 12 months and every year annually. What do I have to do to earn these gifts? I just have to place at least a 50PV or above order consistently for 3 months, 6 months, 9 months and 12 months and my gift will be sent with that month's ER order.

Below are what the standard planned gifts are for consecutive ordering, but that might be switched out with another oil of like value if it is out of stock.

- For 3 consecutive months, the gift is a 5 ml of Peppermint Vitality™ Essential Oil.
- For 6 consecutive months, the gift is a 5 ml of Thieves® Vitality™ Essential Oil Blend.
- For 9 consecutive months, the gift is a 15ml of Melaleuca Alternifolia Essential Oil.
- For 12 consecutive months, the gift is a 5 ml of Loyalty™ Essential Oil Blend. This is a special blend formulated by D. Gary Young exclusively for Essential Rewards members who have loyally ordered for 12 consecutive months and is awarded annually.

That sounds pretty cool to me, but I know there are more ways to get paid shopping in my own store. The next way is by saving on shipping, and while I can already save money on shipping by choosing Essential Rewards, there are more ways to save.

Young Living has two different options for Essential Rewards members who want to save money on pre-paid shipping costs.

The first option is called YL Go, and it costs $59.00 for 12 essential rewards orders and one bonus shipment to be shipped out without any additional cost. Since the cheapest shipping method costs at least $5.99 for 3-8 day delivery, I'm already saving about $18-$20 by choosing this option and I get my order in 2-3 days.

The second option is called YL Go+, and it costs $129 for 12 months of ER shipments and 24 bonus shipments to be shipped out without any additional cost. With this option, I'm already saving about $86-$100 and I still get my order in 2- 3 days.

With either YL Go or YL Go+ I can also choose to expedite my order to overnight by paying an additional $10 per use.

I really like getting paid to shop at my own store, with quality products I can trust, and I'm supporting my family's health at the same time!

Ask Yourself...
Do you like saving money? Did you realize you could transfer buy? How can you use Essential Rewards to support your family's health?

Income Disclosure Statement

The Federal Trade Commission (FTC) makes sure that distributors do not make false or misleading income claims and requires that the income disclosure statement be included when income is discussed for MLMs. So, with all the talk about income and compensation, I thought it would be best to follow FTC rules and include a copy of the Young Living Income Disclosure statement.

You will find a link provided in the bonus material available on the book website, TheBestEO.com for a current, higher quality, color version.

YOUNG LIVING 2017 WORLDWIDE INCOME DISCLOSURE STATEMENT

WORLDWIDE INCOME STATISTICS FOR JANUARY–DECEMBER 2017

WHAT ARE MY EARNING OPPORTUNITIES? This document provides statistical, fiscal data about the average member income and information about achieving various ranks.

YOUNG LIVING MEMBER RANK	PERCENTAGE OF ALL BUSINESS BUILDERS[1]	MONTHLY INCOME[2]				ANNUALIZED AVERAGE INCOME[3]	AVERAGE MONTHS TO ACHIEVE RANK[4]		
		Lowest	Highest	Median	Average		Low	Average	High
DISTRIBUTOR	33.3%	$0	$725	$15	$26	$312	N/A	N/A	N/A
STAR	41.02%	$0	$932	$58	$75	$906	1	12	267
SENIOR STAR	15.66%	$2	$5,531	$193	$235	$2,819	1	19	255
EXECUTIVE	6.62%	$34	$13,210	$425	$502	$6,028	1	25	254
SILVER	2.55%	$229	$29,248	$1,698	$2,088	$25,059	1	32	252
GOLD	0.57%	$1,506	$48,630	$4,541	$5,666	$67,995	2	49	263
PLATINUM	0.18%	$4,375	$90,275	$11,057	$13,872	$166,468	5	58	243
DIAMOND	0.07%	$6,256	$163,387	$27,972	$35,348	$424,178	7	70	251
CROWN DIAMOND	0.01%	$28,492	$231,397	$53,589	$64,477	$773,724	16	85	258
ROYAL CROWN DIAMOND	0.02%	$50,770	$326,334	$132,828	$144,551	$1,734,606	17	97	230

1. Because a member's rank may change during the year, these percentages are not based on individual member ranks throughout the entire year but are based on the average distribution of member ranks during the entire year. Business Builders are members who have personally enrolled at least one other person and does not include Preferred Customers.

2. Because a member's rank may change during the year, these incomes are not based on individual member incomes throughout the entire year but are based on earnings of all members qualifying for each rank during any month throughout the year.

3. This is calculated by multiplying the average monthly incomes by 12. These incomes include income earned from January 1, 2017, through December 31, 2017, but which was paid between February 2017 and January 2018.

4. These statistics include all historical ranking data for each rank and thus are not limited to people who achieved these ranks in 2017. Members who do not make at least one product purchase in the previous 12 months are considered inactive.

The income statistics in this statement are for incomes earned by all worldwide active Business Builder members in 2017. An "active Business Builder" member is a member who made at least one product purchase in the previous 12 months and has personally enrolled at least one person during the lifetime of the member account. The average annualized income for all active Business Builder members in this time was $3,321, and the median annualized income was $684.

Note that the compensation paid to members summarized in this disclosure does not include expenses incurred by members in the operation or promotion of their business, which can vary widely and might include advertising or promotional expenses, product samples, training, rent, travel, telephone and internet costs, and miscellaneous expenses. The earnings of the members in this chart are not necessarily representative of the income, if any, that a Young Living member can or will earn through the Young Living Compensation Plan. These figures should not be considered as guarantees or projections of your actual earnings or profits. Young Living does not guarantee any income or rank success.

Proof In Action – Check The Facts

We have learned how Young Living follows the rules on FDA and Lacey Act compliance and how they spend their money rewarding the people who are consistently ordering or sharing. I've included a list of bullet points from this chapter below.

Compliance, The FDA, & Vague Descriptions

- The FDA doesn't allow Young Living or any independent distributors to make disease claims.
- Young Living cannot claim that an essential oil or product will cure, treat or prevent any disease and can only make Dietary Supplement Claims.
- Young Living can make one of 4 types of Dietary Supplement Claims, Health, Nutritional, Well-Being, and Structure or Function.
- Dietary Supplement Claims have to include the obligatory statement: "This statement has not been evaluated by the Food and Drug Administration. This product is not intended to diagnose, treat, cure, or prevent any disease."

The Lacey Act of 1900

- Originally created to monitor the unlawful sale or possession of plants, fish and wildlife, but was expanded in 2008 to include a wider variety of prohibited plants and plant products.
- Young Living demonstrated integrity by self reporting when they unknowingly violated the law, doing the right thing, even thought they knew that they would

be prosecuted and fined for reporting themselves.
- Young Living is currently the only essential oil company with a Lacey Act Compliance Plan.
- Young Living only sources products from ethical, sustainable sources that are conflict free.

Why Network Marketing Makes Sense

- Word-of-mouth advertising generates five times the sales of paid media advertising.
- People are 90% more likely to buy a product if recommended by a friend.
- Young Living sends thank you checks to people for talking about what they love, educating on products and helping others!
- Would you like to get a thank you check for sharing what you love?

The Accidental Paycheck

- Young Living members frequently get an accidental paycheck for sharing what they love.
- The Young Living Compensation Plan Video https://vimeo.com/106306657

Getting Paid To Shop In My Own Store

- Young Living rewards people with free products when ordering at different price points, and even at intervals for ordering consistently.
- It is easy to save money by transfer-buying toxin laden products from the grocery store to Young Living's awesome toxin-free products and earn free products at the same time.

- There are options on pre-paid shipping that save significant amounts of money.

Income Disclosure Statement

- The FTC requires that the income disclosure statement be included when income is discussed for MLMs.

Young Living has more products than just essential oils. In the next chapter I'll discuss some of the 600+ life-changing products that make up the health lifestyle of Young Living.

CHAPTER 9

Healthy Lifestyle

"Follow your dreams, work hard, practice and persevere. Make sure you eat a variety of foods, get plenty of exercise and maintain a healthy lifestyle."
~Sasha Cohen

Savvy Minerals Makeup

As a guy, my experience with makeup is limited to watching my wife and our oldest daughter enjoy their Savvy Minerals by Young Living™.

Previously, my wife, Carrie, did not like to wear makeup at all, because she didn't like the feeling of having something on her face. She felt like she was suffocating. She also didn't like that the products were made with talc, bismuth, parabens, phthalates, petrochemicals, fetal tissue, nanoparticles, synthetic fragrances or colorants, or cheap synthetic fillers.

When Carrie first heard about the new Savvy Minerals by Young Living™, she was so excited! Not only is there none of the nasty stuff listed above in Young Living products, but they are filled with pure, natural and safe ingredients. Even more, after trying it, she felt like she wasn't wearing anything on her face but looked fabulous!

Savvy Minerals by Young Living are:
- Seed to Seal® verified
- Contain high-quality, color-rich minerals
- Enhanced with Young Living essential oils,
- Aspen bark extract as an all natural preservative
- Mica, a pure earth mineral added for shimmer
- Naturally derived, vegan and vegetarian friendly ingredients (except beeswax in the lipstick)
- Conscientious beauty without compromise

As Young Living is constantly improving and adding more options, the current, Savvy Minerals by Young Living™ Products include:

- 10 Colors of Foundation
- 2 Bronzers and 2 Veils
- 7 Shades of Blush
- 12 Eyeshadow Options
- Eyeliner and 4 MultiTaskers
- Lip Scrub
- 6 Lip Gloss Varieties
- 11 Lipstick Shades
- 10-piece Salon Quality Brush Set
- Essential Oil Infused Misting Spray

Now, I watch my wife joyfully put on makeup, and she looks radiant, and doesn't have to worry about how toxins are affecting her health! She loves the variety, choices, and versatility of the products. She loves experimenting with new colors and methods, and says that the makeup is very forgiving, because you can use the different shades so many different ways.

These wonderful mineral-based makeups can be used on every skin type and skin tone. Women all over the world are raving about the Savvy Minerals Makeup!

Even more wonderful for us, since we know these products are safe, our oldest daughter is now able to use makeup without harming her health. Now, she is also able to experience the joy of using makeup.

Would you like a toxin-free makeup you can trust and looks amazing?

Thieves® Non-Toxic Cleaning & Products

There are so many reasons to like the Thieves® line of products, and I love to use them everywhere in my house. I can't think of a single thing that we don't use Thieves® Cleaner to clean. In my family, we use Thieves® products for laundry, washing dishes, whole house cleaning, cars, wood furniture, and floors. We also take capsules of it, support optimal health, diffuse it, brush our teeth with it, and use it as a hand purifier.

Before I continue, let me take a moment to explain why it's called Thieves®. This is a blend we have due to the tenacity, research and passion of Gary Young as he read about and researched a group of thieves operating during the plague of 1720. These thieves were also perfumers who went around robbing the bodies of the dead, sick, and dying, and thought they would never be caught. They were caught, however, and forced to divulge their secrets, and to everyone's disbelief they found out they were using a blend of essential oils!

When Gary heard about this story, he was intrigued and curious, spending hours at the British Museum and library archives searching stories, but all of his hard work paid off. All of his research led to the amazing Thieves® essential oil blend. Gary brilliantly combined Clove, Cinnamon Bark, Eucalyptus Globulus, Lemon, and Rosemary essential oils to create the Thieves blend.

Modern scientists have analyzed the chemical constituents and benefits of the different oils that make up this blend, and understand why the thieves used that blend long ago. Today we know that Clove is a protector, Rosemary is a balancer, Eucalyptus is an oxygenator, Cinnamon is a purifier, and Lemon is uplifting and invigorating with its wonderful citrus fragrance.

Today, there's a large body of reserach available on the properties and benefits of the components of the Thieves® Essential Oil Blend; in fact, there was even a study done by Weber State University in Ogden, Utah in 1998 that published their results on the Thieves® blend itself.

Besides the Thieves® essential oil blend, the most often used Thieves® product in our house is the Thieves® Cleaner. With eight children, we always have a use for Thieves® Cleaner around our house, from cleaning up spills, potty training, wiping down counters and cleaning crayon and marker off the wall. We have thoroughly tested the Thieves® Cleaner!

Thieves® Cleaner is such a cost saver as well for our family, because instead of having 5 or even 10 different cleaners for the different surfaces in our house, I buy one cleaner, put a capful in a spray bottle and fill the rest with water. For less than a dollar per spray bottle, I have a product that does a better job on windows, counters, floors, toilets, and even furniture than any other cleaners I have used!

On top of that, Thieves® cleaner is made from all-natural plant based ingredients, and I feel totally at peace to give it to my children to clean bathrooms and counters, and even to my two year old to clean the baseboards. I feel safe knowing that this cleaner is not laden with toxins!

Six reasons to use Thieves® Cleaner:

1.   SAFETY - Not having to worry about toxic chemicals around children, pets, and the elderly. Thieves® Cleaner is a toxin-free cleaner derived from plant-based ingredients.

2.   AIR QUALITY - In most cleaning products there are volatile organic compounds that have been associated with multitude of health problems including damage to the liver, kidneys, and central nervous system. Thieves® Cleaner smells great, and is such a joy to use, because I can breathe deeply while I spray it without worrying about toxins in the air.

3.   ENVIRONMENTAL IMPACT - Most cleaners nowadays harm fish, animals, humans and the rest of the environment. Thieves® Cleaner is gentle on fish, animals, humans and earth's ecosystems, and yet is more awesome than any other cleaner I have ever used.

4.   CONVENIENCE - Being able to reduce the number of toxic products in the house and clean everything with just one product is amazingly simple. In my family, we clean an entire bathroom with one spray bottle full of Thieves® Cleaner and two rags. We use a microfiber rag on the mirror, faucets, countertop, shower walls, tub and then toilet, switch rags and clean the floor!

5.   COST - Saving money purchasing one cleaner instead of a multitude is a huge cost savings. Additionally one 14.4 Oz bottle of Thieves® Cleaner gives you 30 bottles of cleaner at less than a dollar a bottle!

6. **SCENT** - Having to suffer a chemical smell in your house when something spills at your party is hard on your guests. When we need to clean up a spill, out comes the Thieves® Cleaner and we get comments on how much they like the scent!

I've spent some time talking about the Thieves® Cleaner product. My admiration for all the Thieves® products is great, and in the last chapter, I will highlight my favorite Thieves® products, that we use throughout our house!

NingXia Red® & Ningxia Nitro™

Although some people call it "Ninja Red," and my friend Sarah even pronounces it, "Knee-sha Red," its actual pronunciation is closer to "Ning-Sha Red." It is made using the wolfberry, otherwise known as the Goji berry from The NingXia Province in China.

Ningxia Red® is an antioxidant rich superfood drink that gives me lots of energy without any funny stuff, crash, or jitters. I know it supports every system in the body, but I love how I feel so energized and alive! I usually drink two ounces of NingXia Red® in the morning and sometimes forget to eat breakfast because I feel so nourished and my brain feels activated. I especially love to drink NingXia Red® after a workout to shorten my recovery time.

Gary Young first heard of the amazing health benefits of this particular species of wolfberry from Dr. Songqiao Chao, a Chinese scientist and Dean of the Science Department of the Beijing Technical University. Dr. Chao was giving a guest lecture at Weber State University in Utah, and while visiting was invited to meet Gary.

As the two of them talked, Dr. Chao became interested in Gary's work with essential oils, and Gary became interested in Dr. Chao's work with wolfberries. According to Dr. Chao's research, due to the fertile, mineral rich soil of the NingXia Province, this particular wolfberry species, *lycium barbarum L*, has significantly greater health benefits than any other kind of wolfberry species in China! As a result, this particular province in China is one of the longevity hotspots in the world, where people live actively into their hundreds.

Gary was excited and found a grower of this particular species in the Elbow Plateau of the NingXia Province, and began importing dried berries. He then combined the wolfberry puree with the other well- known antioxidant rich juices of aronia, pomegranate, cherry, plum and blueberry and added Orange, Tangerine, Lemon, and rare Yuzu essential oils. This truly blessed combination contains powerful compounds, phytonutrients, polyphenols, vitamins and minerals. It is high in the fiber Zeaxanthin, critical amino acids, and polysaccharides, giving you a unique nutritional profile so you don't miss out on any of these vital nutrients.

NingXia Red® is one of my favorite drinks, and rarely does a day go by where I do not drink at least 2 oz of this wonderful tasty goodness! However, NingXia Red® is not the only NingXia product available. I also love the NingXia Nitro™, NingXia Zyng™ and Wolfberry Crisp Bars!

NingXia Nitro™ combines wolfberry seed oil, ginseng, B vitamins, green tea extract, and other select ingredients along with an Energy Blend of essential oils, which includes Black Pepper, Nutmeg, Peppermint, and Spearmint to support cognitive alertness and fitness.

NingXia Nitro™ replaced my morning cup of coffee. It wakes me up in less than 5 minutes, instead of taking about an hour for a cup of coffee!

Vitamins & Supplements

Not all supplements are the same, and here, Young Living once again comes out on top. Recently in the news, the New York State Attorney General's office tested the supplements from 4 major chain stores, and the results found out that up to 90% of the products contained nothing of the substance that they claimed to have in them and instead contained rice and other fillers. What a sad state of affairs when businesses put profit over people!

Young Living is all about the people, and the Seed to Seal® quality promise is throughout the entire company, especially in all the products they produce! That is why Young Living always seeks to go above and beyond, to create an even better product. Sometimes being the best takes a continuous improvement process, being willing to always improve and looking to bring new and higher quality products onto the market, whether it be by changing components, resources or processes.

While Young Living already has high quality supplements, (with the actual ingredients in them), Young Living does research and testing to perform the continuous improvement process with their supplements.

From what I've heard, Young Living tested supplements and found out that it took two weeks and people were only absorbing about 60%. Young Living found out that if they infused the supplements with essential oils, the process drastically improved the body's ability to absorb the vitamins, minerals and nutrients. The new result was that after the first two hours people were already absorbing 80% or more.

After that, Young Living changed its processes to infuse a large portion of its supplements with essential oils, and the people benefit! Now instead of buying a product and using it for two weeks to see any benefit, people start to see benefits from the first day.

When I first tried Young Living Supplements, I noticed the difference right away. One of the first supplements I tried was Young Living's Super B™ vitamin, and I noticed the difference in the first 1/2 an hour. I have tried B vitamins from multiple different sources throughout my time in the military, but the Super B™ vitamin from Young Living, is noticeably different and awesome!

I have had the same experience with every vitamin and supplement I have tried from Young Living. Would you like the same experiences?

Personal Care & Other Products

Young Living has products for every area of your life and everyone in your life.

There are products for men, women, children, babies, athletes, fitness and health, and even weight management.

Men are well taken care of with products that include not only essential oils and supplements but also all of the Shutran™ products, from shaving cream to beard oil, and from deodorant to soap.

Women are provided an entire line of skin care products with the ART® Skin Care System, Savvy Minerals Makeup, facial care products, lotions, moisturizers, soaps, bath gels, body, and hair care products.

The products for children are part of the whole Kid Scents® line which includes a set of pre-diluted essential oil blends for more sensitive skin, toothpaste, shampoo, vitamins, and supplements.

Babies also have an entire line devoted just to them, the Young Living Seedlings™ line, which includes all of your baby and diaper bag needs, including Lavender baby wipes, the OTC labeled Diaper Rash cream, baby oil, baby shampoo and more!

Athletes, fitness and health enthusiasts benefit from the Pure Protein Complete meal supplement, PowerGize™, AminoWise™, NingXia Red®, NingXia Nitro™, essential oil singles for discomfort after workouts, blends like R.C.™ and PanAway®, massage oils, the Active and Fit Kit, and a whole line of vitamins and supplements.

Individuals looking for awesome weight management products love Young Living Slique® products and their annual Slique® challenge which help provide a step in the right direction toward a healthier, happier, self.

Animals & Pets

Animal health was always very important to Gary, and one of his particular loves were horses. Young Living has the largest working draft horse team in the world, and they are incredibly well taken care of and loved. The Young Living Percherons, Draft Horse team has won multiple medals and awards for their training, abilities and appearance, and Gary created multiple animal blends and products to care for these magnificent animals.

Whether for farm animals or pets, Young Living has the entire Animal Scents™ product line to support them all, big or small. Currently, there are 10 products labeled exclusively for animal use, but there have also been multiple books written to help you care for the animals and pets in your life with a variety of Young Living products.

Would you like your furry, feathered and scaled friends to be able to use healthy products too?

Proof In Action – Check The Facts

Living a healthy lifestyle can be a daunting thing without the right company to partner with, but Young Living makes it easy by having products for every area of your life. Take a few minutes to review the benefits of each area.

Savvy Minerals Makeup

- No talc, bismuth, parabens, phthalates, fetal tissue, petrochemicals, nanoparticles, synthetic fragrances or colorants, or cheap synthetic fillers.
- Joyfully put on makeup, look radiant, without worry of toxins affecting your health.
- Enjoy the variety, choices, and versatility of the products.
- Experiment with new colors and methods, with the forgiving makeup that lets you use the different shades in so many different ways.
- Wonderful mineral-based makeups can be used on every skin type and skin tone.
- Women all over the world are raving about the Savvy Minerals Makeup!
- Would you like a toxin-free makeup you can trust and looks amazing?

Thieves® Non-Toxic Cleaning & Products

- Thieves® products for laundry, washing dishes, whole house cleaning, cars, wood furniture, and floors.
- Clean scent loved by family, party guests and friends.

- Modern scientists have analyzed the chemical constituents and benefits of the different oils that make up this blend, and understand why that blend was used.
- Thieves® Cleaner is used all around the house, from cleaning up spills, wiping down counters and toilets to cleaning walls.
- It is safe to use Thieves® Cleaner around children, pets, and the elderly.
- Awesome air quality makes breathing easy without worry of airborne toxins.
- Gentle on fish, animals, humans and earth's ecosystems.
- One non-toxic cleaner replaces all of the cleaners in the house and does a better job.
- Concentrated 14.4 oz bottle makes 30+ bottles of cleaner at less than $1 per bottle.

NingXia Red® & Ningxia Nitro™

- Ningxia Red® is an antioxidant rich superfood drink.
- Is a wolfberry species in China with significant health benefits.
- From a longevity hotspot, where people live actively into their hundreds.
- Combined wolfberry puree with the other well-known antioxidant rich juices of aronia, pomegranate, cherry, plum and blueberry.
- Infused with Orange, Tangerine, Lemon, and rare Yuzu essential oils.
- Contains powerful compounds phytonutrients, polyphenols, vitamins and minerals, and it is high in fiber Zeaxanthin, critical amino acids, and polysaccharides.

- NingXia Nitro™ combines wolfberry seed oil, ginseng, B vitamins, green tea extract, and other select ingredients along with an Energy Blend of essential oils.
- NingXia Nitro™ includes Black Pepper, Nutmeg, Peppermint, and Spearmint to support cognitive alertness and fitness.

Vitamins & Supplements

- Young Living does research and testing to perform the continuous improvement process with their supplements.
- Young Living changed its processes to infuse its supplements with essential oils to increase effectiveness.
- People start to see benefits from Young Living vitamins and supplements on the first day!

Personal Care & Other Products

- Young Living has products for every area of your life and everyone in your life.
- Over 600 products are available for Men, Women, Kids, Babies, Athletes, Fitness and Health, and even Weight Management.

Animals & Pets

- Gary created multiple animal blends and products to care for the Young Living Percherons and other animals.
- Young Living's Animal Scents™ product line supports all animals, big or small.

- Multiple books are available written to help you care for your animals and pets.

In the final chapter I will discuss the scenarios of good, better, best and awesome, to figure out which one is right for you. I will also be sharing some of my favorite products with you, so move along to the last chapter and lets see how you can get started with Young Living!

CHAPTER 10

Getting Your Own

"To get it first is important -
but more important is to get it right."
~Jessica Savitch

Good, Better, Best & Awesome

I have been talking about my favorite essential oil company, Young Living Essential Oils, and I've mentioned the Young Living lifestyle, a way of living a happier and healthier life. The Young Living Lifestyle is where you are able to substitute all the toxin-laden products in your house with products from Young Living that are toxin-free and support your health.

You want to get some of Young Living's amazing products in your life, but how do you get them, and what do you choose? Well, I think my friend Chris Opfer says it best when he says, "It is kind of a Good, Better, Best scenario.

GOOD is as a customer paying retail, because you get great products, and good if you only want to get one single bottle of oil and never want to order again.

BETTER is as a wholesale member, and it's better because you get 24% off everything that Young Living has to offer, think Shoppers Club. You also get other member exclusives and you're all set up to share should you ever choose to do so.

Now the **BEST** option, which is what I do, is as an Essential Rewards member. I took that wholesale membership and I started earning points back on everything I order.

Young Living starts you at 10%, after three months, you go to 20% and eventually you go to 25%. In addition to that, you also get free gifts at 3, 6, 9, and 12 months. The 12 months gift is an awesome Loyalty oil, that you cannot buy otherwise!

In addition to everything you also get free shipping or discounted shipping depending on which program you choose. That's sort of like your Shoppers Club meets your online home delivery meets your cash back credit card, Young Living just does it better!"

My hope is that I have empowered you to make a decision of what's right in your life! Now you need to make a choice about what is right for you.

But wait, I mentioned a fourth choice, **AWESOME**! Awesome is choosing the best option and then not keeping the knowledge to yourself, but sharing what you know and love with others. While you were reading, you probably thought of three friends that would benefit from what you now know. So take it to the awesome level, and share with the three friends or family members you have been thinking about, and you might just get an Accidental Paycheck too!

If you are saying, "This is all great information, but how do I sign up?" Then...

If you **have someone who is sharing with you** about Young Living, go to them and ask them to help you sign them up.

If you **do not have someone sharing with you** about Young Living, I would love to have you on my team! You are welcome to go to the book's website, TheBestEO.com and you will find a signup link there.

My Favorite Products

My favorite Young Living Products for myself and my family include:

- **Single Essential Oils**: Idaho Balsam Fir
- **Additional favorites**: Black Pepper, Copaiba, Frankincense, Goldenrod, Lavender, Sacred Frankincense, Tea Tree, and Peppermint.

- **Essential Oil Blends**: Valor®
- **Additional favorites**: Believe™, Highest Potential™, Humility™, ImmuPower™, Inner Child™, PanAway®, Raven™, Reconnect™, Relieve It™, Shutran™, Thieves®, and White Angelica™.

- **Kits/Collections**: Oils of Ancient Scripture™
- **Additional favorites**: Feelings™, Freedom Release™, Freedom Sleep™, Infused 7™, Raindrop Technique®, and Reconnect™

- **Supplements**: Super B™,
- **Additional favorites**: AgilEase™, CortiStop®, Master Formula™, MultiGreens™, Life 9™, OmegaGize^{3}®, DetoxZyme®, Longevity™ Softgels, Mineral Essence™, and SleepEssence™.

- **Drinks**: NingXia Red®, NingXia Nitro™, and NingXia Zyng™ mixed together!
- **Additional favorites**: AminoWise™, Vanilla Pure Protein™ Complete, Slique® Tea.

- **Massage Oils**: Sensation™
- **Additional favorites**: Ortho Ease®, Ortho Sport®, Relaxation™

- **Snacks**: Wolfberry Crisp™ Bars
- **Additional favorites**: Gary's True Grit® Einkorn Granola, Slique® Bars, and anything made with Gary's True Grit® Einkorn Flour

- **Over The Counter Products**: Cool Azul™ Pain Cream
- **Additional favorites**: Insect Repellant, Lavaderm™ After-Sun Spray, Mineral Sunscreen Lotion SPF 10 & 50, and Thieves® Cough Drops

- **Accessories**: HydroGize™ Water Bottle
- **Additional favorites**: Lantern Diffuser and Desert Mist Diffuser

My family's favorite household and personal care products for a toxin-free lifestyle include:

- **All Purpose Cleaner:** Thieves® Cleaner to wash our dishes, clean our windows, mirrors, counters, furniture, floors, and cleaning up messes.

- **Laundry:** Thieves® Landry Detergent and wool dryer balls with Lemon, Lavender or Purification® essential oils

- **Dishes**: Thieves® Dish Soap to wash dishes.

- **Hand Soap:** Thieves® Hand Soap - Bathrooms, Kitchen, and garage sink.

- **Hand and Body Lotion**: Lavender and Genesis™ Hand & Body Lotion in our bathroom and kitchen.

- **Bathroom favorites include**: Charcoal bar soap, Copaiba Vanilla Shampoo, Copaiba Vanilla Conditioner, Mirah™ Shave Oil, KidScents® Toothpaste, Essential Beauty™ Serum, Thieves® Mouthwash, and Thieves® AromaBright™ Toothpaste

- **Makeup and Skincare**: Savvy Minerals by Young Living™ and all the ART® products, for my lovely wife and oldest daughter.

- **My wife and my teen daughters love**: Progessence Plus™ Syrum, EndoFlex™ Blend, Dragon Time™ Blend, Dragon Time™ and Relaxation™ Massage oils.

- **Products for my children and infant**: KidScents® Shampoo, KidScents® MightyPro™, KidScents® MightyVites™, Seedlings™ Lavender Baby Wipes, and Seedlings™ Diaper Rash Cream

- **My kids' favorite products at Bedtime**: ImmuPro™ tablets, Lavender essential oil, Gentle Baby™ Blend, SleepyIze™ Blend, Dream Catcher™ Blend, and SleepEssence™ gel-caps.

Summary

Well, we finished our walkthrough and found out what is the best essential oil company, answered many questions that pop up when talking about essential oils and Network Marketing companies. Now it is time to review the information and make your decision!

Good, Better, Best & Awesome

GOOD is as a customer paying retail, because you get great products, and good if you only want to get one single bottle of oil and never want to order again.

BETTER is as a wholesale member, you get 24% off everything that Young Living has to offer and you also get other member exclusives and you're all set up to share, should you ever choose to do so.

BEST is what I do as an Essential Rewards member. I took that wholesale membership and I started earning points back on everything I order.

AWESOME is not keeping the knowledge to yourself but sharing what you know and love with others.

Favorite Products

I've listed what my favorite products and my family's favorites are; now it is your turn to figure out what products are your favorites!

Please feel free to visit the book website at TheBestEO. com for a complete list of questions and summaries from all of the Proof In Action sections as a special gift and to see the bonuses available for download.

Thank you for allowing me the privilege of sharing what I've learned. I wish you the very best and happy oiling!

About the Author

Bill Liebich lives in Vail, AZ with his amazing wife and eight wonderful children. He is a former Cisco Network Engineer, retired as a Technical Sergeant from the USAF as a Russian Linguist, and is now the CEO of Living Fully Anointed, LLC.

Bill is known among his peers to have a complex and analytical mind, which easily and systematically sorts through the data to discover the facts, uncovers the truth and exposes the deception. He has a gift for simplifying complex concepts, topics and ideas related to health and natural remedies, and has shared his personal journey to health freedom in ways that resonate with people seeking alternatives to western medicine.

Bill has spent over 15 years researching and studying healthy living using holistic methods, with the past 6 ½ years being devoted to the use of essential oils extensively. There is not one single over the counter or prescription drug in his home. His family of ten has experienced the use of essential oils in many daily life occurrences, emotional stressors, and even several first aid and emergency situations. Spend a day with Bill and within one hour you'll feel like you just got a lifetime of wisdom. He simply loves to share all that he's learned throughout his lifetime of experiences and training.

Bill is a fun family man who loves spending his free time working on home improvements, tinkering in the garage, and working with his hands. He enjoys speed walking and seeing the expressions of joggers as he passes them. Archery is one of his most favorite pastimes. He has split an arrow in twine and is passing his archery skills down to his children. Anyone who has ever met Bill knows Thai food is his absolute favorite cuisine. He and his wife go every week for date night to Luckie's Thai where he never has to order. They see him walk in and alert the cook and then hand him his bill.

The award-winning author travels extensively across the world conducting seminars and workshops to educate individuals and groups on essential oils, and help businesses educate their employees on healthy living strategies to lessen sick days, increase performance and support a more focused and relaxed environment. He is available for delivering keynote presentations; for rates and availability, please contact the author directly at Bill@theBestEO.com.

Testimonials

"There is a common problem in the essential oil marketplace today, too many lies being told, cloaked in smoke and mirrors, making it difficult to find the truth. Bill does and excellent job of identifying the vital information, cuts through the lies, and provides a resource for living a truly healthy life!"

Dr. Olivier Wenker, MD, MBA, DEAA, ABAARM, FAARFM Physician, Author, International Speaker, Scientific Advisor Physician for Integrative, Antiaging, and Regenerative Medicine, Houston, Texas

"Exploring alternative avenues from the mainstream is of great benefit to your health and well-being. Remember that essential components also include nutrition, exercise, lifestyle, attitude, mindset and gratitude. On this journey many questions will arise.

Bill Liebich's *What Is The Best Essential Oil Company? Cutting Through The Lies,* is an essential resource when exploring essential oils. The questions raised in this book will remove all of the guess work and lead you to making informed decisions regarding your well-being. By balancing all aspects of your life, you can Heal Your Health Naturally."

Dr. Stacey Cooper, Award-Winning Author of Heal Your Health, The Healthy Fuels Cookbook, International #1 Bestselling Author of What's Self Love Got To Do With It?, International Speaker, Founder of Lifestyle Balance Solutions, Chiropractor, Teacher, Coach, and Consultant. Brantford, Ontario Canada

"A terrific distillation of the essential oil marketplace! This book is a must-read for knowledge seekers. No longer do you have to comb the web to figure it out on your own. This is your manual for finding the oily lifestyle you want. After reading this book, I wanted to see how prevalent toxins were in my home; I was so surprised! I'm convinced and I no longer have to guess where to buy essential oils."

Frank Kemberling, Pastor of Freedom Fellowship Ministries, Tucson, AZ

"Bill is phenomenal, I love his wealth of knowledge and the way he truly cares about people is fantastic. His spectacular personal testimonials and stories were life-changing for me, and I know they will do the same for you!"

Tammy Goerke, Mentor at ACA Life Mentoring, Lawernceville, Georgia

"This book takes the mystery out of finding the best quality essential oils for my family. As a mom of two, I care about what I am giving my kids. Not only did I find the best company, but I found a recipe for healthy living choices too!"

Gueniviere Chrankshaw, Military Spouse, Stay-At-Home Mom, Holmen, Wisconsin